HEALTH
ASSESSMENT

A MODULAR APPROACH

HEALTH ASSESSMENT

A MODULAR APPROACH

Peggy M. Mayfield, R.N., M.S.N.
Associate Professor
Adult Nurse Practitioner
Harris College of Nursing
Texas Christian University
Fort Worth

Mary Lou Bond, R.N., C.N.M., M.N.
Associate Professor of Nursing
Harris College of Nursing
Texas Christian University
Fort Worth

Marta Askew Browning, R.N., M.S.N.
Assistant Professor of Nursing
Harris College of Nursing
Texas Christian University
Fort Worth

Jane Cooper Evans
Associate Professor of Nursing
College of Nursing
University of Texas at El Paso

McGraw-Hill Book Company

New York   St. Louis   San Francisco   Auckland   Bogotá   Hamburg   Johannesburg   London   Madrid   Mexico
Montreal   New Delhi   Panama   Paris   São Paulo   Singapore   Sydney   Tokyo   Toronto

HEALTH ASSESSMENT: A Modular Approach

3 4 5 6 7 8 9 0   DODO   8 9 8 7 6 5 4 3 2 1

This book was set in Univers Light by Allen Wayne Technical Corp. The editors were Laura A. Dysart and Irene Curran; the designer was Anne Canevari Green; the production supervisor was Jeanne Skahan. The cover was designed by Rafael Hernandez. The drawings were done by Marcia Williams, Boston University Medical Center.
R. R. Donnelley & Sons Company was printer and binder.

Library of Congress Cataloging in Publication Data
Main entry under title:

Health assessment.

    1.   Nursing—Programmed instruction.
2.   Physical diagnosis—Programmed instruction.
3.   Medical history taking—Programmed instruction.
I.   Mayfield, Peggy M.
RT48.H43   610.73   79-18505
ISBN 0-07-041027-5

To Peggy,
with the greatest of
professional respect
and personal affection

Mary Lou
Marta
Jane

CONTENTS

PREFACE

This manual is the cumulative result of our efforts to incorporate physical assessment skills into the curriculum of Harris College of Nursing, Texas Christian University. We are, respectively, an adult nurse practitioner, a nurse-midwife, a pediatric clinical specialist, and a community health nurse with preparation as a clinical specialist in psychiatric nursing. The diversity of our backgrounds, preparations, and approaches to health care soon led us to enlarge our view beyond strict physical examination to the concept of health assessment. This philosophy is represented throughout the materials presented in this manual.

We view health assessment as a more comprehensive approach than physical examination alone and believe that it more accurately depicts the nurse's role in the delivery of health care. We believe that health assessment is an integral part of the nursing process and that professional nurses should be prepared to collect a complete health history and perform a systematic physical and psychological assessment. This data base serves as a basis for planning, implementing, and evaluating nursing care and, when necessary, for referring the client for further evaluation and treatment. Tools and approaches suggested seek to depict the total client situation — physical, psychological, and social — within the context of meaning which it has for the individual client. Thus, this workbook does not isolate the physical examination from the examination of other sectors of the client's life. The individual is viewed as a whole, and assessment is made of the total person.

We feel that students learn best when they are actively involved in the teaching-learning process and when they can select those learning activities most meaningful to them. Therefore, a list of suggested readings, audiovisual materials, and learning activities is presented in each module; each module also includes an annotated Decision Table. From this array of material, students and faculty can select those experiences which best meet module objectives based on the learning style of the student.

Health Assessment: A Modular Approach focuses on the health history and physical and psychological assessment of the adult, with adaptations for the pediatric, geriatric, and obstetric client. Adaptations for four ethnic groups—black, Mexican-American, American Indian, and Oriental—are also included. The flowchart on the inside front cover guides the student through the modules, and annotated decision tables present a variety of optional learning strategies. History and physical assessment forms serve as guides in performing and recording health assessments. Behavioral objectives, pretests and posttests, and evaluation tools for faculty assessment of the student serve as guides for determining mastery of knowledge and skills.

The organization of the instructional modules allows flexibility in that the modules can be taught in a clearly defined physical assessment course, integrated as separate modules throughout a preexisting curriculum, or used selectively to meet specialized needs of a curriculum.

We wish to express our appreciation for the enthusiastic response of students who participated in the pilot study for evaluation of these modules, and to Dean Virginia Jarratt for her support and encouragement.

We are also grateful to Helen Fielden for her patience and endurance in the typing and preparation of the manuscript, and to Richard Swinson, whose investment of time, talent, and ideas contributed much to the format of this manual.

Peggy M. Mayfield
Mary Lou Bond
Marta Askew Browning
Jane Cooper Evans

HEALTH ASSESSMENT

A MODULAR APPROACH

INTRODUCTION

DIRECTIONS FOR THE STUDENT

These instructional modules are designed as a guide to assist you in learning a thorough and systematic approach for health assessment, to be used in conjunction with appropriate texts and media. The authors have designed this manual to maximize student participation in decision making regarding appropriate learning experiences which will meet module objectives. This workbook is not intended to be used without supervision and validation by a qualified instructor.

Texts and media have been suggested for each module, but comparable references and media may be selected. Your instructor or school will determine the learning activities to be completed within the modules and the levels of mastery to be attained on the Pretests, Posttests, and assessment performance guides.

A modular approach was selected to enable you to make preliminary preparation, utilizing a variety of learning methods prior to classroom or clinical practicum with the faculty. Each module is similar in approach. You may find the flowchart on the inside front cover helpful as a guide for the use of each module. As you begin each module, carefully read its introduction and objectives. Overall objectives for each module are similar. These are listed in this Introduction. However, specific Prerequisite Objectives and Terminal Objectives are given in each module. The Prerequisite Objectives in most of the modules pertain to anatomy and physiology of the pertinent unit of study. Take the Pretest and score it. If your score is inadequate, review anatomy and physiology before continuing the module. Please note that the Pretest does not prepare you for the Posttest.

Read the suggested references and view the suggested media. Review the Vocabulary and look up any unfamiliar terms. The Vocabulary is divided into descriptive and diagnostic terminology.

Next, you will want to make an assessment card or cue card to guide you in performing the history and physical examination of the body system.

You are now ready to take the Posttest. If your score is satisfactory, you are ready to proceed to the clinical component, which may be performed in a skills laboratory or clinical setting. If you need additional review or wish to pursue specific interests, you will find helpful suggestions in the annotated Decision Table in each module. A master Decision Table of references used throughout the workbook is given in this Introduction.

As you perform an assessment of an adult friend or client, use the adult health history and assessment forms provided in each module to record the data. in assessment of the pediatric, geriatric, and obstetric client, use the adult form along with the appropriate adaptation guidelines. Ethnic variations should be noted as appropriate to the system assessed. At the end of each assessment form, you are asked to report recommendations for reevaluation or referral for follow-up of abnormal findings. These recommendations become criteria upon which the instructor may evaluate the following behaviors:

1. The ability to differentiate the normal from the abnormal
2. The ability to identify nursing needs and problems of clients
3. The ability to establish priorities for the nursing needs of clients
4. The ability to make decisions regarding reevaluation, referral, and future plans for follow-up

An Instructor's Guide for Evaluation of Student Performance is included in each module. This guide allows you to clarify the assessment techniques which will be evaluated by the instructor. It also ensures consistency in expectations and evaluation among instructors when several may be involved in evaluating students. The guide may further help you with organization and sequence of examination.

Upon completion of all modules, perform a complete health assessment using your cue cards. Organize the complete assessment so as to minimize your client's position changes and energy expenditure. An abbreviated model adult history, physical examination form, and newborn assessment form are included in the Appendix for your use in a complete health assessment.

OVERALL OBJECTIVES

Upon completion of this manual you are expected to be able to:

1. Take a health history, with an assessment form as a guide, using appropriate branching questions.
2. Perform a systematic physical and psychological assessment, using an assessment form as a guide.
3. Describe the anatomical differences between the newborn, child, and adult that will be of significance to the examiner.
4. Demonstrate variations of technique used in examination of the child.
5. Describe age-related changes that occur with the geriatric client.
6. Describe anatomical and physiological alterations occurring throughout the prenatal, intrapartal, and postpartal phases.

7. Describe variations in approach used in collecting and interpreting data obtained from various ethnic groups.

8. Describe variations in the physical characteristics that may occur among ethnic groups.

9. Record the data obtained from the health assessment, using correct medical terminology.

10. Differentiate between findings which are within normal limits and those which need further evaluation or represent abnormalities.

SUGGESTED REFERENCES

Alexander, Mary, and Marie Brown: *Pediatric History Taking and Physical Diagnosis for Nurses,* McGraw-Hill, New York, 1979.

Bates, Barbara: *A Guide to Physical Examination,* Lippincott, Philadelphia, 1979.

OR

Malasanos, Lois, et al.: *Health Assessment,* Mosby, St. Louis, 1977.

Caird, F. I., and T. G. Judge: *Assessment of the Elderly Patient,* Pitman, California, 1977.

OR

Saxon, Sue V., and Mary Jean Etten: *Physical Change and Aging,* The Tiresias Press, New York, 1978.

Mahoney, Elizabeth A., et al.: *How to Collect and Record a Health History,* Lippincott, Philadelphia, 1976.

MASTER DECISION TABLE

If . . .	Then . . .
You need help with history taking and suggestions for branching questions	Wasson, John, et al.: *Common Symptom Guide,* McGraw-Hill, New York, 1975.
You prefer well-illustrated material	Prior, John A., and Jack Silberstein: *Physical Diagnosis,* Mosby, St. Louis, 1977.
	Delp, Mahlon H., and Robert T. Manning: *Major's Physical Diagnosis,* Saunders, Philadelphia, 1975.
You need a comprehensive reference on growth and developmental changes through the life cycle	Murray, Ruth B., and Judith P. Zentner: *Nursing Assessment and Health Promotion through the Life Span,* 2d ed., Prentice-Hall, Englewood Cliffs, N.J., 1979.
You desire in-depth coverage (for the advanced student)	DeGowin, Elmer L., and Richard L. DeGowin: *Bedside Diagnostic Examination,* Macmillan, New York, 1976.
You seek concise material regarding the history and physical examination	Fowkes, William C., and Virginia K. Hunn: *Clinical Assessment for the Nurse Practitioner,* Mosby, St. Louis, 1973.

MASTER DECISION TABLE (continued)

If . . .		Then . . .
	⇒	Gillies, Dee Ann, and Irene B. Alyn: *Patient Assessment and Management by the Nurse Practitioner,* Saunders, Philadelphia, 1976.
You desire alternative health assessment texts	⇒	Sana, J. M., and R. D. Judge (eds.): *Physical Appraisal Methods in Nursing Practice,* Little, Brown, Boston, 1975.
	⇒	Sherman, J. L., and Sylvia Fields: *Guide to Patient Evaluation,* Medical Examination Publishing Company, Flushing, N.Y., 1974.
You desire a concise book on geriatrics, with a helpful table on the physiological effects of aging	⇒	Adams, George: *Essentials of Geriatric Medicine,* Oxford, New York, 1977.
You seek a collection of references on gerontology which contains several scales for the functional assessment of the elderly client	⇒	Brantl, Virginia M., and Sister Marie Raymond Brown (eds.): *Readings in Gerontology,* Mosby, St. Louis, 1973.
You desire an in-depth coverage of physiology of aging	⇒	Timiras, P. S.: *Developmental Physiology and Aging,* Macmillan, New York, 1972.
You seek a thorough text on the normal aging process, deviations from the normal, and nursing implications	⇒	Burnside, Irene M.: *Nursing and the Aged,* McGraw-Hill, New York, 1976.
You desire additional pediatric references	⇒	Burness, Lewis A.: *Manual of Pediatric Physical Diagnosis,* Year Book, Chicago, 1972.
	⇒	Chinn, Peggy L.: *Child Health Maintenance,* Mosby, St. Louis, 1974.
	⇒	Chinn, Peggy L., and Cynthia Leitch: *Child Health Maintenance: A Guide to Clinical Assessment,* 2d ed., Mosby, St. Louis, 1979.
You need to review the Denver Developmental Screening Test	⇒	Frankenburg, William K., et al.: *Denver Developmental Screening Test Manual,* University of Colorado Medical Center, Denver, 1970.
You desire information on cultural and biological diversity and health care.	⇒	*Nursing Clinics of North America,* **12**(1), March, 1977.
	⇒	Branch, Marie Foster, and Phyllis Perry Paxton (eds.): *Providing Safe Nursing Care for Ethnic People of Color,* Appleton-Century-Crofts, New York, 1976.

MODULE 1

HEALTH HISTORY

The data base for any client is composed of three main sections — the health history or client profile, the results of the physical examination, and the laboratory and diagnostic test results. This module features collection and recording of the health history, the foundation upon which the two remaining components of the data base rest.

Except for the additional section, Brief Guidelines for Students, the format for this module is similar to that of the succeeding modules. To complete the module, you may wish to follow the general instructions presented by the flowchart on the inside front cover in combination with the specific instructions given in the Suggested Activities section which follows. You are to complete the required activities and pass the Posttest before proceeding to the skills laboratory for demonstration of technique.

The section of the health history titled Review of Systems (ROS) is covered in more detail in each module and in the Appendix. It is attached here to indicate that a detailed ROS is normally a part of the health history, but the detailed review will not be the major focus of this module.

If you have any difficulty completing this module, consult your instructor.

PREREQUISITE OBJECTIVES

You should be able to:

1. Cite the purposes of an interview.
2. Describe the factors that promote an effective milieu for interviewing.
3. Describe the stages of an interview.

4. Identify techniques which facilitate and give direction to the interview.
5. Identify techniques which block effective communication.
6. Discuss the role of nonverbal behavior in the communication process.
7. Discuss the impact of social distance on the interview process.
8. Identify ways in which expectations for outcome on the part of both client and interviewer affect the interview process.
9. Describe techniques which facilitate communication with the elderly.
10. Cite special considerations to be made in the implementation of a pediatric interview.
11. Discuss special problems in establishing communication lines with the adolescent.
12. Discuss the impact on the interviewing process of cultural differences between the client and interviewer.

TERMINAL OBJECTIVES

Upon completion of this module you are expected to be able to:

1. Describe the significance of the data base in health assessment.
2. List the component parts necessary to compile a data base (health assessment).
3. Define *chief complaint.*
4. Describe the method of eliciting and recording data for the chief complaint.
5. List the data to be included in the record or history of the present illness.
6. Discuss the components which must be included in an analysis of a symptom.
7. Identify the components of a family history and its relationship to the total health assessment.
8. Identify the components of a social history and its relationship to the total health assessment.
9. Identify the components of a past medical history and its relationship to the total health assessment.
10. Describe the review of systems (ROS) and its relationship to the total health assessment.
11. Describe the way in which data for the ROS is organized and recorded.
12. Cite adaptations in the health assessment data base to be made for the pediatric client.
13. Discuss cultural factors that may influence the progress of the interviewing process.
14. Discuss characteristics of an elderly client which the interviewer must consider in collecting a health history.
15. Conduct an interview for collection of a health history, using a data base.
16. Using appropriate terminology, record the data obtained in an interview.

GUIDELINES FOR STUDENTS

The inclusion of this section is a departure from the format used in these modules, and an explanation is in order. A number of sources were used in compiling the material for this module. In no one source did the authors find the following information, which is inherently understood by experienced, successful interviewers. Portions of this material were touched upon in various sources, but nowhere was this information located in one easily accessible reference. Therefore, we are including our "helpful hints" here in the hope that they will prove useful to you as you begin history-taking interviews.

Hint 1

You will note that the Health History and Assessment section of this module is quite long and extremely detailed. It is designed in this manner to enable the student to see the type, depth, and scope of information required within each category or area of concern. In the Appendix you will note an abbreviated or skeletal history form. This form is more common and will be seen frequently in clinical settings. Judgment must be exercised in selecting the type of form to be used in a given situation. The preferred form will depend upon a number of variables.

Generally speaking, a detailed health history form will be used in clinical settings or agencies that seek to provide the client with comprehensive health supervision encompassing the following features:

1. Long-term contact
2. Health-maintenance services
   a. Primary prevention
   b. Anticipatory guidance to defuse potential problem areas
   c. Early intervention in developing problems
   d. Health education

3. Treatment or referral for treatment
4. Supervision and reinforcement of treatment program
5. Continuity and coordination of care
6. Coordination, supervision, and reinforcement of the rehabilitation program
7. Involvement of the family in the planning and implementation of the client's health care program

Settings in which these characteristics exist include independent nursing practices, visiting nurse associations, community health agencies, group practices of clinical specialists, outpatient clinics, family practice clinics, and mental health clinics.

The abbreviated form is more appropriate for inpatient settings such as hospital units, specialty clinics, offices of specialists, industrial health settings, and emergency rooms, where contact is relatively short and not designed for health maintenance and long-term behavioral change. In using the abbreviated form, bear in mind that indications of problems in a given area will require a more detailed interview and appropriate branching questions to explore problems or concerns of the client more fully.

Hint 2

You must develop your own style as an interviewer. This style should be based on a thorough understanding of interviewing techniques and approaches, but adapted in a way that reflects your own personality. It will become your "personal touch" in the therapeutic relationship. No two interviewers will approach and conduct an interview in the same manner. An attempt to adopt someone else's style as your own will cause the client to suspect a "phony," and responses will be altered accordingly.

During the preparation period preceding the interview session, each interviewer must decide how to phrase or state questions to obtain the necessary information. Seldom will such questions appear verbatim on the health history form. Statements and questions on the health history form are there as prompters for the interviewer. Individual differences in client personalities should determine the approach selected, and questions should be presented in the way deemed most appropriate for "this" client in "this" situation. You will *gradually* (not instantly) develop a highly flexible repertoire. This will come only with repeated practice and contact with many different client personalities and problems.

Hint 3

Ideally, the *initial* health history should be taken in one scheduled interview session of about 1 to $1\frac{1}{2}$ hours; however, our present culture is oriented toward the "illness-treatment" concept of health care. It is important to keep this in mind since this is also likely to be the client's concept of the health care system. This orientation will explain why most clients will first contact you when they are ill or concerned about some abnormality. In this situation, it is best to obtain the chief complaint, history of present illness, and other related history, and then provide for examination and treatment and reappoint for follow-up. On the follow-up visit, a more complete health history may be taken or an additional time may be scheduled for such an endeavor. No client can comprehend the reason for the acquisition of data on a lengthy form when ill and interested in conveying to the professional only information relevant to the present distress.

Hint 4

The recent focus of consumer demand on health maintenance and preventive health care has not yet altered the illness-treatment orientation of most clients. Their initial contact with the health history form may place them on unfamiliar ground, and once the interviewer strays away from the now familiar history of present and past illnesses, the client's anxiety level may increase until it reaches the point of resistance and outright hostility. If this point is reached, the relationship is irreparably damaged. This situation need *never* occur. Remember you are on different "wavelengths." The client is thinking, "illness-treatment." You are viewing the gamut: prevention of illness, early detection and intervention, treatment, rehabilitation leading to a state of high-level wellness.

Cue the client in! Change the client's wavelength and enlist active cooperation. It is difficult to play the game without knowing the rules or how to score a goal. Remember, it's the client's health and health history. You are being employed to help interpret this individual's data.

Try the following:

1. Make sure you introduce yourself, give your position or title, and tell the client how you are related to the agency. (It's good if you can also give this data in writing so clients can contact you later if they become anxious, have second thoughts, or need to supply additional information.)

2. Schedule a specific time to conduct the interview. Explain that this will require 1 to $1\frac{1}{2}$ hours of the client's time. This information helps the individual do some planning so that he or she can more comfortably participate in the interview without worrying about being late for work or other activities.

3. Explain that since you will be seeking to provide the client with comprehensive *health* supervision, you will need to collect a broad range of data that will form a profile of the individual as a person. Such a profile can be developed only by exploring current health status, past health and medical history, personal habits and preferences, and social and psychological aspects of the individual's life.

This comprehensive data collection is needed before

a. Potential problem areas or factors predisposing to illness may be identified.

b. Present health problems, either overt or covert, may be identified.

c. Intervention and follow-up appropriate to the client's unique personality and situation can be planned and implemented.

d. Areas in which the client may need health instruction can be determined.

Explain that all areas will be explored, since all can affect the client's health status.

4. Instruct the client that at any point in the interview he or she may request you to clarify the relevance of any questions you are asking, and that the client may refuse to answer any questions felt to be inappropriate.

5. Tell the client that all information collected is considered privileged (strictly confidential) and may be used only by other professionals involved in the client's care. (If you can tell who these are, do so.) No information can be released to relatives, employers, or insurance companies without written consent.

6. Explain that you will review with the client data collected during the interview and allow time for evaluation, clarification, and correction of misinterpretations.

7. Explain that, based on this review, you will identify any current health needs together. Those identified as most important by the client will receive top priority for action.

This approach allows the client maximum control and freedom in the relationship. It sets the tone of the relationship as one designed to serve and meet individual needs. In this "show," the client can become the "star" and to a great extent control the situation.

Since individual contact time is limited in many clinical settings, and since client conditions vary, collection of the health history in one interview session may be undesirable if not impossible. Several interviews or patient contacts may be required to obtain the necessary information. Indeed, such data collection will continue throughout the life cycle of the relationship. As the relationship grows and trust is established, more information will be shared and new insights formed. As appropriate, the data base must be altered to reflect this knowledge.

Be patient—don't rush it. After all, it took you more than 18 years to develop a health history of your own. How would you feel if you had to reveal all in 1 hour?

Hint 5

In evaluating the data collected, the emphasis should be on assessing *patterns* of health behavior. Seldom is one piece of data alone significant, nor can any piece of data be judged significant if taken out of the context of meaning it has for the client.

Hint 6

The tremendous variety in background and personality in both health professionals and clients is almost incomprehensible to contemplate. You will never treat a client who is exactly like you in every respect. Some clients will be more like you than others, and with these rapport will be more easily established. Other clients will come from an environment and value orientation totally alien to yours. It is the responsibility of the nurse to deliver health care to all, both those like and those unlike the care giver. For this reason, you will note a number of optional readings related to the concept of culture and specific cultural groups. These are suggested to stimulate your awareness of the vast gulfs that, at times, separate human beings—gulfs that cultural blindness often prohibits us from seeing. Unless the nurse is aware that such differences may exist, it will be virtually impossible to establish a relationship of trust with the client or to plan care which is acceptable and can be implemented in the client's own environment.

SUGGESTED ACTIVITIES

Read

Bates, Barbara: *A Guide to Physical Examination,* Lippincott, Philadelphia, 1979 (sections on health history for adult and pediatric clients).

OR

Malasanos, Lois: *Health Assessment,* Mosby, St. Louis, 1977 (sections on adult, pediatric, and geriatric histories).

Alexander, Mary, and Marie Brown: *Pediatric History Taking and Physical Diagnosis,* McGraw-Hill, New York, 1979 (section on the history-taking interview).

"Patient Assessment: Taking a Patient's History," *American Journal of Nursing,* February: 293–324 (1974).

View

The Health History, Part 2, Interview for the Health History, Blue Hill Educational System videotape (IVT 19) 26 min.

Review

Vocabulary list

Student performance assignment

1. Complete Pretest with mastery.
2. Complete readings and related assignments above.
3. Complete Posttest with mastery.
4. Gather equipment
   a. Tape recorder and tape
   b. Pens and pencils
   c. Data-base form
5. Select a friend for collection of the data in the data-base interview. Explain the procedure.
6. Interview the friend. Tape-record the interview.
7. Record the information on the data-base form prior to listening to the tape.
8. Listen to the tape. Evaluate your technique in collecting information, and correct the information as necessary.
9. Submit the data base, or reinterview and submit an improved data base to your instructor for evaluation and feedback.

PRETEST

Answer questions in the space provided. You may check your answers using the answers in the back of this book. Mastery of test material is required before continuing with this module.

1. A number of purposes exist for conducting a client interview in the course of health care delivery. Name at least *three* of these.

2. Establishment of a climate conducive to effective interviewing is essential for the health professional. List at least *three* techniques which aid in establishing such a climate.

3. Several activities are listed below. On the line to the left of each activity, place the letter which identifies the phase of the interview in which you would expect to find the activity. The four phases of an interview are: preparation (*P*), initiation (*I*), direction (*D*), and termination (*T*).

   a. _____ Introduction of the interviewer to the client.

   b. _____ Discussion of future plans for treatment.

   c. _____ Formulating questions which fulfill the objectives of the interview.

   d. _____ Explaining to the client what is expected during the interview.

   e. _____ The interviewer guides the interview by questions.

   f. _____ A statement by the interviewer that the interview will soon be drawing to a close.

   g. _____ The professional greets the client by name.

   h. _____ The interviewer formulates objectives for the interview.

   i. _____ The interviewer explains to the client the ways in which the information collected will be used.

   j. _____ The interviewer summarizes the data and gives the client the opportunity to make corrections as necessary.

4. Verbal responses of the interviewer to the client may be grouped into five major categories:

   a. Evaluative or judgmental

   b. Hostile or defensive

   c. Reassuring (false reassurance)

   d. Probing or challenging the client's motives

   e. Understanding or accepting

   In the space to the left of the following interviewer responses, identify the type of response given to the client.

   Client: "You know that Dr. Jones? He's totally incompetent. He doesn't know what he is doing. These medicines he prescribed are not doing me any good at all."

   a. _____ "I understand how hard it is for you when you are sick. Just be patient. Dr. Jones is a fine doctor and he knows what he is doing. You'll be feeling much better in just a few days."

    b. _____ "You don't seem to be telling me everything. You are obviously quite upset — surely it's not just about the medications."

    c. _____ "You seem to be upset. You mention having problems with the medication prescribed by Dr. Jones. Can you tell me a little more about the problems you are having with it?"

    d. _____ "You mustn't get so upset. It's not good for your condition. Don't you think you are being a bit irrational? You have only been on the medication for 24 hours."

    e. _____ "Dr. Jones is the finest doctor practicing in this area. You probably haven't been following his instructions."

5. The following group of techniques are called _____

    _____ communication.

    a. Stating personal experiences or opinions

    b. Value judgments

    c. Defensiveness

    d. Use of clichés and stereotyped responses

    e. Challenging client's motives

Indicate whether the following statements are *true* (T) or *false* (F).

6. _____ Observation of client behavior during the interview is selective and may be influenced by conscious and unconscious responses of the interviewer.

7. _____ Data obtained by observation is limited to that triggered by visual stimuli.

8. _____ Verbal responses of the client are the most important responses to be considered by the interviewer.

9. _____ Nonverbal behavior is always under the conscious control of the client.

10. _____ Nonverbal behavior includes not only typical mannerisms of the client but also observable physiological responses such as blushing.

11. _____ Commenting on the client's patterns of nonverbal behavior may encourage the client to express his or her inner experience more fully.

12. _____ Open-ended questions are used in the interview to limit the interviewer's control over client communication.

13. _____ Silence is to be avoided in the therapeutic interview.

14. _____ Clients often filter out responses that they consider to be shameful or feel that the interviewer will find unacceptable.

15. _____ The tactful interviewer will change the subject when the client is about to be overwhelmed by emotion.

16. _____ Crying by the client indicates that the interview is out of the interviewer's control.

17. _____ A client will often control anger toward the health professional.

18. _____ A client who has a strong need to maintain independence may minimize symptoms for fear of being ordered to bed.

19. _____ The guiding principle of open-ended interviewing is that the clinician exerts the least amount of authority or direction necessary to obtain data.

20. _____ Clients always consult health professionals about health problems.

21. _____ The client's expectations concerning the interview have less effect than the interviewer's.

22. _____ An active role on the part of the interviewer and a passive role on the part of the client elicit the greatest client satisfaction.

23. _____ A good interviewer will relieve the client of responsibility for the outcome of the therapeutic relationship.

24. _____ A "helping" interview is usually structured, utilizes a predetermined tool, and avoids delving deeply into the personality structure.

25. _____ In an information-gathering interview, the client chooses what to speak about and is allowed to speak freely.

26. _____ Selective inattention is used more often by the client than by the interviewer.

27. _____ To evaluate a child, it is best if parent and child can be interviewed both individually and together.

28. _____ Children are not to be considered reliable in describing symptoms. The parent is the preferred source for such information.

29. _____ Information obtained from parents may be biased, as they will seek to present themselves and their child in a good light.

30. _____ The most important element in establishing a climate for effective interviewing is establishing trust between client and professional.

31. _____ The same or similar information will be elicited by all health *professionals* interviewing the client.

32. _____ A stubborn resistive silence on the part of the client will usually evoke reciprocal anger in the novice interviewer.

33. _____ Abruptly changing the subject or cutting the client off is a method by which the interviewer reduces his or her own anxiety.

34. _____ Adolescent clients tolerate silence well.

35. _____ When the client's verbal and nonverbal behavior don't agree, confronting the client with this fact is a technique which may be used by the interviewer.

36. _____ The interviewer must maintain an awareness of visual or auditory changes in an elderly client that will require adjustments in interviewing techniques.

37. _____ In interviewing the elderly client, the interviewer may find that a relatively long pause will occur between question and response as the client sorts through a vast store of accumulated mental data to give a complete response.

38. _____ All necessary information about a client is collected in one interview.

39. Social distance (cultural or class differences) between interviewer and client often block communication. Cite at least *three* reasons for this.

40. Awareness of several special techniques aid in facilitating an interview with an elderly client. A list of several techniques is listed below. Classify each of these as *helpful* or *not helpful* in the space provided.

    a. _____ Speak loudly since hearing may be impaired.

    b. _____ Sit face-to-face or where the elderly client can maintain eye contact with you.

    c. _____ Block the client's attempts to reminisce as he or she is fixated on past.

    d. _____ Address the client as "Grandpa" or "Grandma" to create a more personal climate for the interview.

    e. _____ Accept the information given as accurate without cross-checks or validation.

VOCABULARY

accepting or understanding response
baseline data
body language
chief complaint
chronology
clarification
client
closed questions
communication blocks
confrontation
facilitative
false reassurance
defensive or hostile response

health history
interview
nonverbal behavior
observation
open-ended questions
perception
reflective response
review of systems (ROS)
selective inattention
sensory overload
summarization technique
territoriality
verbal behavior

DECISION TABLE 1-1

If . . .		Then . . .
You wish to review an excellent book on interviewing with a programmed-learning format, illustrations, examples of what to do and what not to do, and some detailed examples of interviews		Froelich, Robert E., and Marian F. Bishop: *Clinical Interviewing Skills*, Mosby, St. Louis, 1977.

DECISION TABLE 1-1 (continued)

If . . .		Then . . .
You need to review a general introduction to communication and basic interviewing	⟹	Baer, Ellen D., et al.: "How to Take a Health History," *American Journal of Nursing,* 1190-1192 (July, 1977).
	⟹	Gillies, Dee Ann, and Irene B. Alyn: *Patient Assessment and Management by the Nurse Practitioner,* Saunders, Philadelphia, 1976 (medical history and psychosocial assessment).
	⟹	Malansanos, Lois, et al.: *Health Assessment,* Mosby, St. Louis, 1977 (interview).
	⟹	Murray, Ruth, and Judith Zentner: *Nursing Concepts for Health Promotion,* 2d ed., Prentice-Hall, Englewood Cliffs, N.J., 1979, pp. 61-98.
You wish to view media	⟹	*The Nurse-Patient Interaction,* Concept Media.
	⟹	*Techniques of Therapeutic Communication, Program 4,* Concept Media.
	⟹	*Blocks to Therapeutic Communication, Program 5,* Concept Media.
	⟹	*Effective Listening,* Trainex (PC 293).
	⟹	*Verbal Barriers to Communication,* Trainex (PC 294).
	⟹	*Non-Verbal Barriers to Communication,* Trainex (PC 295).
You need to review basic interviewing and basic interviewing techniques, interviewing the child, interviewing the family, patient responses to illness, and expectations of the health care system that affect the interview	⟹	Enelow, Allen T., and Scott N. Swisher: *Interviewing and Patient Care,* Oxford, New York, 1972, pp. 3-49, 102-161, 177-206.
You need to glean further understanding of the client's responses to illness and its impact on the interview, classification of interview responses, and samples of responses	⟹	Bernstein, Lewis, et al.: *Interviewing: A Guide for Health Professionals,* Appleton-Century-Crofts, New York, 1974.
You desire an excellent discussion of stages of an interview, techniques for directing an interview, and blocks to effective therapeutic communication (examples given)	⟹	Becknell, Eileen P., and Dorothy M. Smith: *System of Nursing Practice,* Davis, Philadelphia, 1975, pp. 35-59.
You wish some techniques for interviewing the elderly	⟹	Hogstel, Mildred: "Communicating with the Elderly," *Caring,* 14-15 (February-March, 1977).

DECISION TABLE 1-2

If . . .		Then . . .

You seek a detailed explanation of sociological data and as a source for branching questions (this is an excellent reference, as it explains the rationale for the data collected) ⟹ Francis, Gloria, and Barbara Munjas: *Manual of Social-Psychologic Assessment,* Appleton-Century-Crofts, New York, 1976, pp. 1-103.

For comparison, you wish to read another general overview of techniques of obtaining client history which includes samples of data recorded properly ⟹ Fowkes, William C., and Virginia K. Hunn: *Clinical Assessment for the Nurse Practitioner,* Mosby, St. Louis, 1973 (patient interview).

⟹ Mahoney, Elizabeth, et al: *How to Collect and Record a Health History,* Lippincott, Philadelphia, 1976.

You wish another view of baseline data ⟹ Becknell, Eileen P., and Dorothy M. Smith: *System of Nursing Practice,* Davis, Philadelphia, 1975, pp. 35-59.

You seek a comparison of an open-ended and a direct-question approach to obtaining a history ⟹ Bernstein, Lewis, et al.: *Interviewing: A Guide for Health Professionals,* Appleton-Century-Crofts, New York, 1974, pp. 97-109.

You need to gain an understanding of culture and its effect on the formation of a working nurse-patient relationship ⟹ *Ethnicity and Health Care,* NLN Publication 14-1625, 1976.

⟹ Hongladarom, Gail C., and Millie Russell: "An Ethnic Difference—Lactose Intolerance," *Nursing Outlook* (December, 1976).

⟹ Kluckhohn, Florence: "Dominant and Variant Value Orientations," in Pamela Brink (ed.), *Transcultural Nursing: A Book of Readings,* Prentice-Hall, Englewood Cliffs, N.J., 1976.

⟹ Leininger, Madeleine: "Cultural Diversities of Health and Nursing Care," *Nursing Clinics of North America,* **12**(1): 5-18 (March, 1977).

⟹ Leininger, Madeleine: *Nursing and Anthropology: Two Worlds to Blend,* Wiley, New York, 1970.

⟹ Murray, Ruth, and Judith Zentner: *Nursing Concepts for Health Promotion,* Prentice-Hall, Englewood Cliffs, N.J., 1979, pp. 272-298, (culture) 382-436, (religion) 437-476.

⟹ Overfield, Theresa: "Biological Variation—Concepts from Physical Anthropology," *Nursing Clinics of North America,* **12**(1):19-26 (March, 1977).

DECISION TABLE 1-2 (continued)

If . . .		Then . . .
	⟹	Taylor, Carol: "The Nurse and Cultural Barriers," in Barnard Hymovich and Martha Underwood (eds.), *Family Health Care,* McGraw-Hill, New York, 1973, pp. 119-127.
You need information on a client who is black	⟹	Jackson, Jacquelyn Johnson: "The Black Lands of Gerontology," in Marie R. Brown (ed.), *Readings in Gerontology,* Mosby, St. Louis, 1973, pp. 78-97.
	⟹	Jacques, Gladys: "Cultural Health Traditions: A Black Perspective," in Marie Foster Branch and Phyllis Perry Paxton (eds.), *Providing Safe Nursing Care for Ethnic People of Color,* Appleton-Century-Crofts, New York, pp. 115-123.
	⟹	McLaughlin, Clara J.: *Black Parents Handbook,* Harcourt Brace Jovanovich, New York, 1976.
	⟹	White, Earnestine H.: "Giving Health Care to Minority Patients," *Nursing Clinics of North America,* **12**(1):29-31 (March, 1977).
You need information on a client who is Chinese	⟹	Chow, Effie: "Cultural Health Traditions: Asian Perspectives," in Marie Foster Branch and Phyllis Perry Paxton (eds.), *Providing Safe Nursing Care for Ethnic People of Color,* Appleton-Century-Crofts, New York, 1976, pp. 99-112.
	⟹	"Health Care of Chinese in America," *Nursing Outlook,* 245-249 (April, 1973).
	⟹	Louis, Theresa Tsung: "Explanatory Thinking in Chinese Americans," in Pamela Brink (ed.), *Transcultural Nursing: A Book of Readings,* Prentice-Hall, Englewood Cliffs, N.J., 1976, pp. 240-246.
	⟹	White, Earnestine H.: "Giving Health Care to Minority Patients," *Nursing Clinics of North America,* **12**(1):37-39 (March, 1977).
You are seeking information about an American Indian client	⟹	"Caring for the American Indian Patient," *American Journal of Nursing,* 91-94 (January, 1977).

DECISION TABLE 1-2 (continued)

If . . .   **Then . . .**

⟹ Joe, Jennie, et al.: "Cultural Health Traditions: American Indian Perspectives," in Marie Foster Branch and Phyllis Perry Paxton (eds.), *Providing Safe Nursing Care for Ethnic People of Color,* Appleton-Century-Crofts, New York, 1976, pp. 81-98.

⟹ Kniep-Hardy, M., and M. Burkhardt: "Nursing the Navajo," *American Journal of Nursing,* **7**(1):95-96 (January, 1977).

⟹ McCauley, M.A.: "Indian Nurse Considers Cultural Traits," *American Nurse,* **7**(5):5, 15 (May, 1975).

⟹ Mealy, Shirley, and Robert Kane: "Factors That Influence Navajo Patients to Keep Appointments," *Nurse Practitioner,* 18-22 (March-April, 1977).

⟹ Polacca, Kathryn: "Ways of Working with the Navahos Who Have Not Learned the White Man's Ways," in Adina Reinhart and Mildred D. Quinn (eds.), *Family Centered Community Nursing,* Mosby, St. Louis, 1973, pp. 61-71.

⟹ Primeaux, Martha H.: "American Indian Health Care Practices," *Nursing Clinics of North America,* **12**(1): 55-65 (March, 1977).

⟹ Saland, J., et al.: "Navajo Jaundice: A Variant of Neonatal Hyperbilirubinemia Associated with Breast Feeding," *Journal of Pediatrics,* **85**(2):271-275 (August, 1974).

⟹ White, Earnestine Huffman: "Giving Health Care to Minority Patients," *Nursing Clinics of North America,* **12**(1):35-37 (March, 1977).

You need information on a client who is Spanish-speaking ⟹ Baca, J.E.: "Some Health Beliefs of the Spanish Speaking," in Adina Reinhart and Mildred D. Quinn (eds.), *Family Centered Community Nursing,* Mosby, St. Louis, 1973, pp. 72-77.

DECISION TABLE 1-2 (continued)

If . . .		Then . . .
	⇒	Dorsey, Pauline, and Herlinda Jackson: "Cultural Health Traditions: The Latino/Chicano Perspective," in Marie Foster Branch and Phyllis Perry Paxton (eds.), *Providing Safe Nursing Care for Ethnic People of Color,* Appleton-Century-Crofts, New York, 1976, pp. 41-80.
	⇒	Gaitz, Charles, and Judith Scott: "Mental Health of Mexican-Americans: Do Ethnic Factors Make a Difference?" *Geriatrics* (November, 1974).
	⇒	Hymovich, Debra P., and Martha B. Underwood: *Family Health Care,* McGraw-Hill, New York, 1973, pp. 128-148.
	⇒	Martinez, Ricardo Arguijo: *Hispanic Culture and Health Care,* Mosby, St. Louis, 1978.
	⇒	Rubel, A. J.: "Concepts of Disease in the Mexican-American Culture," *American Anthropologist,* **62**:793-814 (1960).
	⇒	White, Earnestine Huffman: "Giving Health Care to Minority Patients," *Nursing Clinics of North America,* **12**(1):32-35 (March, 1977).
	⇒	Wilson, Hollys, and Jose Heinert: "Los Viejitos: The Old Ones," *Journal of Gerontological Nursing,* 19-25 (September-October, 1977).
You have Mexican-American clients who use the services of a folk healer, this may promote understanding	⇒	Kiev, Ari: *Curanderismo: Mexican American Folk Psychiatry,* Free Press, New York, 1968.

POSTTEST   The following questions may be answered *true* (T) or *false* (F). You must answer all questions correctly before you proceed to the laboratory.

1. _____ In recording the name of the client, the first, middle, and last names should be used.
2. _____ Recording of the client's social security number (SSN) aids in a more accurate identification of the client.

3. ____ Recording of identifying data is not necessary when the client is seen only once.
4. ____ *CC* stands for chronic complaint.
5. ____ The CC of a client who is not ill may be a request for health screening.
6. ____ The CC is a summation, in the professional's words, of the client's purpose for requesting health care.
7. ____ The present illness section of the health history describes the chief complaint and is a chronological story of symptoms related to that complaint.
8. ____ In describing a symptom, the practitioner notes that the client's symptoms began two days *PTA,* which means posttraumatic accident.
9. ____ It is helpful to have the client point to the exact location of the pain and trace its course on his or her body rather than relying on a verbal description alone.
10. ____ The adjectives *dull, aching, throbbing,* and *squeezing* may be used to define the *quality* of pain.
11. ____ Clarification by the interviewer will be necessary when the client describes the quantity of pain as "a lot."
12. ____ The interviewer should refrain from asking clients what makes a symptom worse, as this question will only cause clients to focus on all their discomforts, many of which will be totally unrelated to the chief complaint.
13. ____ Negative findings are not noted in the health history.
14. ____ The purpose of the past health history is to identify all major past problems of the client.
15. ____ Data concerning the follow-up of past hospitalizations or illnesses unrelated to the chief complaint are not recorded.
16. ____ It is essential to ask clients about nonprescription drugs they may be taking, which they may not consider to be medications.
17. ____ Information concerning family history is collected only in relation to maternal and paternal grandparents, parents, spouse, and children.
18. ____ The ROS portion of the history consists of information regarding the past and present health of each of the client's body systems.
19. ____ If no symptoms exist in the system being reviewed, the interviewer simply records *negative* under that system.
20. ____ The interviewer should restrict his or her questions to physical data and concerns. Family life is not within the scope of inquiry unless initiated by the client.
21. ____ Eliciting a history of a recent divorce from a client would cause the practitioner to view such a client as a high risk for disease.
22. ____ Cultural factors influence only the socioeconomic portion of the data.
23. ____ Daily habit patterns are explored to determine practices which facilitate or destroy health.

24. _____ The client and the practitioner may not be concerned over the same findings in the data base.

25. _____ The nurse should focus all efforts toward treating the health problems considered to be most severe and pressing, even if they are unrelated to the chief complaint of the client.

26. _____ An adequate recording of data under the system eyes would be ''client wears glasses.''

27. _____ An adequate recording of data under back would be ''denies pain, stiffness, limitation of movement, disc disease.''

28. _____ An adequate exploration of data concerning the client's education would be reflected in the note, ''states he is smart enough.''

29. _____ An example of a chief complaint is, ''I came for my Pap smear.''

30. _____ Questions cannot be asked appropriately nor answers interpreted correctly unless the practitioner understands both his or her own cultural context and the client's.

HEALTH HISTORY AND ASSESSMENT

Health History Form

Identifying data

Client's name_____ Age _____ Birth date _____

Sex _____ Place of birth _____ Social security no. _____

(Married women) Maiden name _____

Husband's full name _____

(Child)   Parent or guardian _____

Current address _____

_____

Phone number at which you can be reached: Business _____

Home_____   Other _____

Health insurance: Policy _____

Policy number _____

Religious preference _____

Source of information for data _____

Chief complaint:

History of present complaint:

Previous Medical History

1. Record of illness

Name of disease or disorder	Inclusive dates (onset to cessation)	Treatment administered	Treating physician and place of treatment	Residual effects or limitations caused by illness
Measles				
Rubeola				
Rubella				
Mumps				
Chickenpox				
Whooping cough				
Scarlet fever				
Diphtheria				
Polio				
Rheumatic fever				
Frequent tonsillitis				
Sinus trouble				
Venereal disease				
Syphilis				
Gonorrhea				
Herpes				
Other				
Cancer				
Heart disease				
Stroke				
High blood pressure				

1. Record of illness (continued)

Name of disease or disorder	Inclusive dates (onset to cessation)	Treatment administered	Treating physician and place of treatment	Residual effects or limitations caused by illness
Diabetes				
Epilepsy				
Hernia rupture				
Prostate trouble				
Allergies				
Hay fever				
Tuberculosis				
Kidney trouble				
Migraine headaches				
Arthritis				
Ulcer				
Stomach trouble				
Anemia				
Sickle cell anemia				
Hepatitis				
Paralysis				
Bleeding tendency				
Vein trouble				
Infantile genetic defect				
Retardation				
Nervous breakdown				

1. Record of illness (continued)

Name of disease or disorder	Inclusive dates (onset to cessation)	Treatment administered	Treating physician and place of treatment	Residual effects or limitations caused by illness
Emotional illness				
Severe injury or accident				
Broken bones				
Burns				
Pneumonia, URIs				
G-6-PD deficiency				
Blood transfusions				
X-rays				
Hospital admissions				
Other				

2. Medication history

Name of drug	Dosage ordered	Dosage taken	Duration of therapy (dates)	Reason for therapy	Effect	Side effect	Last evaluated by M.D.
Prescription drugs							
Nonprescription over the counter							

2. Medication history (continued)

Name of drug	Dosage ordered	Dosage taken	Duration of therapy (dates)	Reason for therapy	Effect	Side effect	Last evaluated by M.D.
Hallucinogens (marijuana, LSD, "speed," other)							
Other							

Patterns of Health and Preventive Health Care Practices

I. Description of usual state of health

II. Routines or regimens followed to maintain health and prevent illness
(For example: BSE, daily oral hygiene, special diets, etc.)

III. Reasons health care usually sought

IV. Symptoms that indicate need for health care

V. Health care practitioners utilized by client and family

Type of practitioner	When last seen	Reason
Neighbor		
Friend		
Native or ethnic practitioner		
Spiritual healer		
Pharmacist		
Chiropractor		
Physician M.D.		
Physician D.O.		
Nurse		
Dentist		
Psychologist		
Psychiatrist		
Nutritionist		
Physical therapist		
Other		

VI. Immunization history

Type of immunization	Dates		Unusual reaction following
Diphtheria			
Pertussis			
Tetanus toxoid			
Tetanus antitoxin			
Polio: Salk			
Sabin:			
Types 1, 2, 3			
Trivalent			
Measles: Rubella			
Rubeola			
Mumps			
Tuberculin skin test:	Pos.	Neg.	
PPD			
Tine			
BCG			
Smallpox			
Influenza			
Swine flu			
Typhoid			
Rabies			
Other			

VII. Corrective appliances

Appliance	Onset of use	Reason for corrective appliance	Date last evaluated by health care personnel
Glasses/contacts			
Dentures			
Hearing aid			
Braces on teeth			
Brace on extremity			
Prosthesis			

VIII. Personal habits

A. Dietary patterns

1. Description or sample of typical daily meal plan:

   Snacking pattern _____

   _____

   _____

   Use of vitamins _____

   _____

   _____

2. Special likes or dislikes _____

   _____

   _____

3. Medical restrictions on diet _____

   _____

   _____

4. Religious restrictions on diet _____

   _____

   _____

5. Impairment in ability to feed self, or mechanical difficulties in chewing food _____

   _____

6. Would you consider yourself a slow eater _____? fast eater _____?

7. Difficulty ingesting milk — lactose intolerance (may be present in Hispanic, oriental, and American Indian clients): _____

8. Would you consider your appetite good? Yes _____ No _____

9. Do you usually eat meals with others _____? alone _____?

10. (Pediatric) Age at which drank from cup _____

    Age at which fed self _____

11. (Infant) Formula _____

    Solid food _____ Names of foods presently taken

    _____

    _____

    Breast-fed _____ Frequency _____

    Length of time on each breast _____

12. Beverages consumed

Name of beverage	Cups per day	Effect	Effect of withdrawal

13. Usual weight _____ Recent gain/loss _____

    Amount _____ Most you have ever weighed _____

    When_____

B. Elimination

    1. Frequency of bowel elimination _____

       Stool color _____ Stool consistency (hard/soft) _____

       Discomfort passing stool _____

       Routines used to maintain bowel habits _____

    2. Frequency of voiding _____

       Quality of stream _____ Color of urine _____

       Amount of urine _____ Difficulty voiding _____

       (Pediatric) Toilet-trained _____ What age _____

       If toilet-trained, does child have accidents _____

       How often _____ When _____

C. Patterns of sleep

    1. Number of hours (24-hour period) _____

       Time usually go to bed _____

    2. Pattern of sleep _____

    3. Frequency of rest periods or naps _____

    4. Disturbances in falling asleep or maintaining sleep _____

    5. Bedtime rituals _____

       Nightmares or dreaming patterns _____

       (Pediatric) If nightmares or sleep disturbances, what action taken by

       parent _____

    6. Number of pillows used _____ Where placed _____

    7. Number of times wake up _____ Why _____

D. Exercise

    1. Amount of exercise per day _____

    2. Limitation of movement _____

    3. Special exercises or exercise programs _____

       _____

E. Sexual behavior

1. Age of onset of sexual activity _____

2. Presently sexually active _____

3. Sexually active with more than one partner _____

4. Homosexual experiences _____

5. Are present sexual patterns and practices satisfying _____

_____

_____

6. Methods of birth control used _____

_____

7. Other sexual habits or unusual sexual experiences (rape, incest, etc.)

_____

_____

8. Male

a. Age at the time of development of

hair on chest _____

hair on face _____

voice change _____

increase in size of genitalia _____

b. Frequency of nocturnal emissions _____

c. Difficulty with maintaining erection or premature ejaculation _____

_____

9. Female

a. Age of development of axillary hair _____

Breast buds _____

b. Age at menarche _____

c. Difficulty experiencing climax _____

d. Frequency, volume, duration of menstrual flow _____

_____

_____

e. Difficulty at midcycle or during periods_____

_____

_____

f. Age at onset of menopause _____

g. Physiological and emotional changes experienced during menopause

_____

_____

h. Date of last Pap smear _____

i. History of vaginal infections _____

j. Childbearing history

Pregnancy	Inclusive dates	Type of birth (live birth, miscarriage, stillbirth)	Prenatal care	Type of delivery	Complications of pregnancy or delivery

F. Tobacco history

Present tobacco use _____ What is used (cigarettes,

cigars, pipe)_____

How much used per day _____Symptoms related to tobacco use

_____

Pattern of use throughout day _____

Smoked in past _____ Pattern _____

Number of cigarettes per day _____ Date of withdrawal _____

Other uses of tobacco _____

G. Alcohol history

Utilization of alcohol _____

Beverages consumed (beer, wine, grain alcohol, etc.)_____

Pattern of usage _____

Consumption — glasses per day _____

Side effects _____

Alcohol-related problems (DWI, auto accidents) _____

Ever treated for alcoholism _____

H. Nervous habits (nail biting, hair twisting, finger drumming, etc.) _____

_____

I. Description of activities in typical day:

Developmental History

This section may be used with any client if data is available, but is a *must* for the pediatric client.

Prenatal history of mother

1. Health during pregnancy _____

2. Number of months prenatal care received during pregnancy _____

3. History of illness, accidents, or hospitalizations during pregnancy_____

_____

_____

4. Medications taken during pregnancy (name, dosage, reason, and month of pregnancy) _____

_____

_____

5. X-rays during pregnancy _____

6. Blood type of mother _____ father _____ client _____

7. Did pregnancy go to term _____

Natal history of client

8. Any problems during labor _____

_____

9. Type of delivery _____

10. Type of anesthesia used _____

11. Baby's (client's) condition at birth _____

_____

12. Weight at birth _____

13. Length of hospital stay _____

14. Were infant and mother discharged at same time _____

15. Any history of cyanosis/jaundice, convulsions, or deformities _____

_____

16. Apgar score _____

17. Weight loss during hospital stay: Actual weight loss _____

Percent of weight loss _____

18. Any history of feeding problems _____

_____

_____

Developmental milestones

19. Age rolled over _____

20. Age first sat alone _____

21. Age crawled _____

22. Age stood alone _____

23. Age walked _____

24. Age talked: Monosyllables _____ Complete words _____

Phrases _____ Sentences _____

25. Eruption of teeth _____ Dentition _____

26. Results of DDST/Press _____

_____

27. Nervous habits (thumb sucking, tics, tantrums, etc.) _____

_____

28. Description of temperament

29. Description of present developmental achievements

Family History

1. Present nuclear family

Names of members	Relationship to client	Age	Occupation	Education	Status of health	If deceased, date and cause of death

2. Client's general description of family
("How would you describe your present family?")

3. Description of roles and responsibilities of family members
("Does wife work?" etc.)

4. Family activities

5. Goals of family

6. Special problems experienced by family

7. Description by client of family's response to stressful situations

8. Observation of interviewer of relationships

   a. Spouse and client _____

      _____

   b. Father and client _____

      _____

   c. Mother and client _____

      _____

   d. Sibling and client _____

      _____

   e. Other _____

      _____

9. Problems with family violence, if any
(Child abuse, wife battering, incest, physical acting out during arguments?)

10. Marital history

Marriage	Duration	Children (names)	If divorced, complete this section		
			Reason for termination	Custody of children	Reaction of child to divorce

a. Client's description of present marriage _____

_____

b. Recent stresses on marriage _____

_____

c. Description of relationship with in-laws _____

_____

d. If children, any problems in child rearing _____

_____

11. Family of origin (extended family—if different from nuclear family)

Names of family members	Rela-tion-ship	Present age	Occupa-tion	Educa-tion	Level of educa-tion	Present state of health	Past ill-ness or chronic condition	If deceased, date and cause of death
Original family (parents, brothers, sisters)								
Maternal family (grandparents, aunts, uncles)								

11. Family of origin (extended family—if different from nuclear family)

Names of family members	Relationship	Present age	Occupation	Education	Level of education	Present state of health	Past illness or chronic condition	If deceased, date and cause of death
Paternal family (grandparents, aunts, uncles)								

a. Brief description of childhood (include problems, adjustments, times of happiness, and feelings about childhood)

b. Brief description of adolescent years (see above)

Socioeconomic History

1. Occupation

a. Present job _____

b. Description of duties of present employment _____

_____

c. Number of days worked per week_____

d. Number of hours worked per week _____

e. Job history (from first employment to present, including military service)

Place of employment	Job title	Duties	Reason for termination

f. Future employment goals _____

_____

2. Family income

a. Classification of family income (per year)

Below $5,000   _____ $16,000 to $20,000   _____

$5,000 to $10,000   _____ $21,000 to $30,000   _____

$11,000 to $15,000   _____   Above $30,000   _____

b. Frequency of paycheck _____

c. Sources of family income _____

_____

_____

d. Method used by family to allocate funds _____

Do family members have allowances _____

Does family make frequent use of credit _____

e. Is income adequate to meet expenses   Yes _____No _____

f. Unusual family expenses or debts_____

g. Methods of payment for health care _____

h. Medical and hospital insurance _____

3. Housing

a. Client's description of and feelings about neighborhood (include services available in neighborhood and distance from health care facility)

b. Client's brief description of and feeling about home

Additional data: Own _____ Rent _____ Length of time in present

home _____ Number of rooms _____ Number of bedrooms _____

Sleeping arrangement_____

State of repair _____

Type of water supply _____ Type of heat _____

Refrigeration _____ Type of toilet facilities _____

Presence of electricity _____ Phone _____ Presence of flies, rodents,

mosquitoes, etc. _____ Health and safety hazards _____

c. History of moves or changes of geographic location

4. Education

a. Educational history

School attended	Type of school	Grade level	Dates	Description of progress	Degree or certificate earned

b. Attitude toward school (what is liked, disliked)

c. Self-enrichment or continuing education:

5. Transportation

Own car _____ Age of car _____ State of repair _____

Friend or family car available for use _____

Utilization of public transportation _____

Use of seat belts and safety devices_____

Does client drive? Yes _____ No _____

6. Recreation

a. Amount of vacation time allotted per year _____

b. Amount of vacation time taken _____

c. History of vacations, including foreign travel:

d. Amount and use of leisure time (hobbies, sports, etc.):

e. (Pediatric) Play activities of client (games, place of play, frequency):

Playmates (number and ages):

7. Cultural background

a. Ethnic group _____

b. Languages presently spoken _____

c. Native language _____

d. Native state _____

e. What place is considered "home" _____

f. Description of changes from cultural or ethnic group of origin

8. Religion

a. Name of church or religious group _____

b. Currently active: Yes _____ No _____ describe activity_____

_____

_____

c. Length of time a member of present religious group _____

d. Brief description of basic beliefs of group with which client agrees

9. Interpersonal relationships and community activities

a. Availability of and relationships with friends

b. (Pediatric) Playmate availability and relationships

c. Community activities

Club and organizational membership	Duration of membership	Function of group	Offices or responsibilities

d. Family, friends, or groups that offer support in times of stress

e. (Adolescent/young adult) dating patterns

Review of Systems

1. General _____
2. Skin _____
3. Head _____
4. Eyes _____
5. Ears _____
6. Nose and sinuses _____
7. Mouth and throat _____
8. Neck _____
9. Respiratory system (thorax and lungs) _____
10. Cardiovascular system _____
11. Gastrointestinal system _____
12. Genitourinary system _____

13. Reproductive system _____

14. Musculoskeletal system _____

15. Central nervous system _____

16. Endocrine system _____

17. Hematopoietic system _____

Student_____

INSTRUCTOR'S GUIDE FOR EVALUATION OF STUDENT PERFOR-MANCE

To evaluate student performance, it is suggested that the instructor observe a 10-minute interview of a client conducted by the student. Performance during this interview may be evaluated in conjunction with a completed history submitted by the student.

Behaviors evaluated	Yes	No	Remarks
1. Prepares general objectives for interview			
2. Selects a site conducive to interview (private, minimum interruptions)			
3. Assures comfort of client			
4. Introduces self to client			
5. Obtains or clarifies client's name			
6. Extends basic courtesies to client (handshake, offer of coffee, request to be seated)			
7. Begins interview with request for chief complaint, using open-ended questions such as, "Tell me how things have been going"			
8. After obtaining complaint, explains purpose of further data collection, identifies data as privileged information, and explains use to be made of data			
9. Is tactful in eliciting personal data			
10. Proceeds to history of illness, follows order indicated by client's focus			
11. Phrases questions in language easily understood			
12. Makes questions simple and brief			
13. Starts with open-ended questions and proceeds to more precise questions or branching questions as indicated			
14. Uses verbal and nonverbal communication to assure client that he or she is functioning adequately			
15. Makes eye contact with client, but avoids staring			
16. Uses touch, if indicated			
17. Controls own distracting body language			

Behaviors evaluated	Yes	No	Remarks
18. Appears relaxed and attentive			
19. Avoids use of blocking techniques			
20. Uses facilitative techniques in directing interview (uses at least five types)			
21. Uses appropriate terminology to record data			
22. Asks branching questions concerning analysis of a symptom, including:			
a. Onset			
(1) Date of onset			
(2) Manner of onset			
(3) Precipitating or predisposing factors			
b. Characteristics			
(1) Character			
(2) Location and radiation			
(3) Intensity or severity			
(4) Timing			
(5) Aggravating and relieving factors			
(6) Associated symptoms			
c. Course since onset			
(1) Incidence			
(2) Progress			
(3) Effect of therapy			
23. Records data collected under ROS in the following order:			
a. Pain or discomfort in organs of system			
b. Functional disturbances of system			
c. Illnesses involving system			
d. Diagnostic test used to identify malfunction in system			
24. Data recorded under chief complaint:			
a. Is brief and concrete			
b. Is restricted to one or two symptoms and includes duration			
c. Uses client's own words in quotation marks			

Behaviors evaluated	Yes	No	Remarks

25. Record of present problem includes:
  a. Elaboration of chief complaint
  b. History of present problem
  c. Description of present status of problem
  d. Symptom analysis
  e. Summary of all significant positive and negative factors related to problem			

26. Interviewer warns client that conclusion of interview is approaching			
27. Summarizes for client significant data collected; gives client a chance to validate, clarify, or change information			
28. Makes general remarks about possible courses of action based on data; allows client to define and offer alternatives			
29. Concludes interview with some statement indicating likelihood of future contacts with client or plans for care of client			

Instructor_____ Date_____

MODULE 2

EXAMINATION TECHNIQUES AND GENERAL OVERVIEW

In this module, emphasis will be placed on the purposes for health assessment. The module will provide an introduction to the fundamental skills needed in making an assessment of the client's health status. You will be introduced to the evaluation of growth and developmental levels, nutritional status, a description of body types, the equipment used in physical examination, four main techniques used in physical examination, methods of obtaining the vital signs, and the development of a general description of the client. Proficiency in these skills and in the collection of a health history will enable you to proceed with the more detailed study of the components of health assessment which follow in succeeding modules.

The goal of health assessment, as presented by the authors in this workbook, is identification of health practices and functions, and differentiation of those which are within normal limits from deviations which may require further evaluation and referral. This workbook does not prepare you to diagnose disease. You will be expected to use the findings of the health assessment as baseline data for supervising the progress of health status over an extended period, identifying client problems requiring further evaluation, planning for client teaching and anticipatory guidance, monitoring effects of prescribed medical treatments and rehabilitation measures, and developing nursing-care plans tailored to meet the needs of the individual client.

You will note that there is no Pretest for this unit. The Decision Table will assist you in acquiring the knowledge necessary to pass the Posttest. Consult your instructor if clarification of material is needed.

The authors are glad to have you with us as you participate in the acquisition of techniques in this and in successive modules.

TERMINAL OBJECTIVES

Upon completion of this module you are expected to be able to:

1. Define health assessment.
2. Cite five reasons for performing a health assessment.
3. Identify the components of a health assessment.
4. Discuss the patterns of growth and developmental change throughout the life cycle.
5. Identify major developmental tasks for the infant (birth to 1 year), the toddler (1 to 3 years), the preschooler (3 to 5 years), the school age child (6 to 12 years), the adolescent (12 to 18 years), the young adult (18 to 45 years), middle adulthood (45 to 65 years), and late adulthood (65 years and over).
6. Discuss the significance of the Apgar score in evaluating the newborn.
7. Discuss the use of the Denver Developmental Screening Test (DDST) in assessment of the preschool child.
8. Perform a DDST and present the results for evaluation.
9. Discuss the following methods for assessing nutritional status of clients:
   a. Dietary surveys (24-hour recall, 3-day food-intake record)
   b. Height and weight comparison
   c. Skin-fold measurements
   d. Physical examination
10. Describe the characteristics of the following types of body builds:
    a. Sthenic — mesomorph
    b. Hypersthenic — endomorph
    c. Hyposthenic or asthenic — ectomorph
11. Define physical assessment.
12. Identify the instruments and equipment used in conducting a physical examination and give examples of use for each.
13. Describe the five major techniques used in conducting a physical assessment — inspection, palpation, percussion, auscultation, and olfaction.
14. Demonstrate the use of these five techniques in obtaining an overview of a client.
15. Identify vital or cardinal signs.
16. Discuss the physiology of temperature, pulse, respiration, and blood pressure and the interrelationships that exist between them.
17. Identify factors which affect the vital signs (e.g., biological rhythm, anxiety, exercise).
18. Identify the normal ranges for T, P, R, and BP in children and adults.
19. Describe factors to be taken into consideration when obtaining vital signs on children.
20. Cite factors which influence the method selected for obtaining temperature by the oral, axillary, or rectal route.

21. Discuss the relationship between the size of the BP cuff and the accuracy of the BP reading.
22. Demonstrate the correct technique for obtaining vital signs (TPR, BP).
23. Describe the relationship that exists between health and weight in healthy clients.
24. Obtain the weights of an adult and a child. Report findings in both pounds and ounces and kilograms and grams.
25. Obtain the height or length of a child and an adult. Report findings using centimeters.
26. Describe the relationship among head circumference, chest circumference, length, and weight in the infant and child.
27. Obtain head and chest circumference measurements of an infant and a child. Report findings in centimeters.
28. Explain the use of percentile standards in evaluating the growth of infants and children.
29. Identify the elements to be included in the general description or brief overview of the client.
30. Given an assessment form, collect and record findings using correct terminology.

SUGGESTED ACTIVITIES

Read

Bates, Barbara: "The Physical Examination of the Adult—An Overview" and "The General Survey," *Physical Examination,* Lippincott, Philadelphia, 1979.

OR

Malasanos, Lois, et al.: "Introduction," "Developmental Assessment," "Nutritional Assessment," and "General Assessment," *Health Assessment,* Mosby, St. Louis, 1977.

Chapters on physical assessment and assessment of vital signs in a fundamentals in nursing textbook.

OR

Wolff, LuVerne, et al.: *Fundamentals of Nursing,* Lippincott, Philadelphia, pp. 284-322 (1979).

Alexander, Mary M., and Marie Scott Brown: "Screening Tests: Common Measurements and Developmental Tests," *Pediatric History Taking and Physical Diagnosis for Nurses,* McGraw-Hill, New York, 1979.

Frankenburg, William K., et al.: *Denver Developmental Screening Test Manual,* University of Colorado Medical Center, Denver, 1970.

Murray, Ruth Beckmann, and Judith Proctor Zentner: *Nursing Assessment and Health Promotion through the Life Span,* 2d ed., Prentice-Hall, Englewood Cliffs, N.J., 1979. (Each chapter contains a list of developmental tasks to be accomplished at each age plus a wealth of other materials. Students may use this book as a resource to develop growth-and-development cue cards.)

View

Temperature, Pulse, and Respiration, Trainex filmstrip with sound (371).
Blood Pressure: Use of Equipment, Trainex filmstrip with sound (101).
B/P Physiology of a Vital Sign, Program 1, Trainex filmstrip with sound (PC 310).
B/P Physiology of a Vital Sign, Program 2, Trainex filmstrip with sound (PC 311).
Assessing Respirations, Concept Media slides with sound.
Abe Ravin, *The Clinical Significance of the Sounds of Korotkoff,* Merck, Sharpe, and Dohme
   audio cassette with text, 1972, 30 min.

Student performance activities

Attend class where your instructor will identify and demonstrate the use of the
following in physical assessment.

1. Ruler and tape measure (centimeter and inch)
2. Cotton-tipped applicator stick
3. Drapes
4. Gloves
5. Gown
6. Examining table
7. Lubricant
8. Ophthalmoscope
9. Otoscope
10. Penlight
11. Percussion (reflex) hammer
12. Safety pin
13. Scales (infant and adult)
14. Stethoscope
15. Sphygmomanometer (aneroid and mercury)
16. Sphygmomanometer cuffs (regular, thigh, pediatric, and infant)
17. Thermometer (rectal, oral, and electronic)
18. Tongue depressor
19. Tuning fork
20. Vaginal speculum
21. Watch with second hand
22. Langes calipers

Attend class or skills lab where your instructor will demonstrate the method of conducting a Denver Developmental Screening Test. Equipment needed—Denver
Developmental Screening Kit containing

   tennis ball
   eight colored blocks
   a rattle
   a bell

a pencil

a bottle

raisins

red wool

DDST manual and forms for recording

After completing suggested readings, viewing suggested audiovisuals, attending demonstrations in class or skills lab, and a period of practice, complete the Posttest and return to the skills laboratory for final evaluation of your performance.

VOCABULARY

Apgar score
antipyretic
apical pulse
apnea
auscultation
asthenic
basic four food
  groups
BP (blood pressure)
bradypnea
bradycardia
cardinal signs
Celsius
centimeter
conduction
convection
developmental delay
developmental tasks

diastolic
dyspnea
ecotmorph
endomorph
eupnea
evaporation
Fahrenheit
febrile
fever
grams
hypersthenic
hypertension
hyposthenic
hypotension
inspection
kilogram
Koratoff sounds
lysis

mesomorph
ounce
palpation
percentile standards
percussion
pound
pulse
pulse pressure
pyrexia
radial pulse
radiation
sthenic
systolic
TPR
tachycardia
temperature
vital signs

DECISION TABLE 2-1

If . . .		Then . . .
You wish some additional help with growth and development	⟹	Erikson, Erik H.: *Childhood and Society*, Norton, New York, 1963.
	⟹	"The Middle Years," *American Journal of Nursing*, 993-1024 (June, 1975).
	⟹	"Staying Well While Growing Old," *American Journal of Nursing*, 1334-1354 (August, 1978).
	⟹	Stevenson, Joanne Sobol: *Issues and Crises During Middlescence*, Appleton-Century-Crofts, New York, 1977.
	⟹	Sutterly, Doris, and Gloria Donnelly: "Table 3-3: Directions of Growth Changes Throughout the Life Cycle," *Perspectives in Human Development*, Lippincott, Philadelphia, 1973.

DECISION TABLE 2-1 (continued)

If . . .		Then . . .
	⇒	"The Young Adult—A Special Feature," *American Journal of Nursing,* **76**(8): 1272–1289 (August, 1976).
A more in-depth discussion of vital signs is desired	⇒	*Assessing Vital Functions Accurately,* Intermed Communications, Pennsylvania, 1977, pp. 15–32.
Further information on blood pressure measurement is sought	⇒	Laneour, Jean: "How to Avoid Pitfalls in Measuring Blood Pressure," *American Journal of Nursing,* 773–775 (May, 1976).
You are curious about temperature regulation in the newborn	⇒	Porth, Carol M., and Leone E. Kaylor: "Temperature Regulation in the Newborn," *American Journal of Nursing,* 1691–1693 (October, 1978).
You want to understand the development of fever	⇒	Davis-Shorts, Jean: "Mechanisms and Manifestations of Fever," *American Journal of Nursing,* 1874–1877 (November, 1978).
You are interested in recent research indicating the possibility of ethnic variation of blood pressure	⇒	Harburg, Ernest, et al.: "Skin Color, Ethnicity, and Blood Pressure I: Detroit Blacks," and "Skin Color, Ethnicity, and Blood Pressure II: Detroit Whites," *American Journal of Public Health,* 1177–1188 (December, 1978).
	⇒	Tyroler, H. A., and Sherman James: "Blood Pressure and Skin Color," *American Journal of Public Health,* 1170–1172 (December, 1978).
Additional discussion of the general inspection of the client is desired	⇒	Prior, John, and Jack Silberstein: *Physical Diagnosis,* Mosby, St. Louis, 1977, pp. 54–62.
You don't know what an Apgar score is	⇒	Korones, Sheldon: *High Risk Newborn Infants,* Mosby, St. Louis, 1976, pp. 53–58.
You desire additional information on assessment of nutrition in childhood	⇒	Pipes, Peggy: *Nutrition in Infancy and Childhood,* St. Louis: Mosby, 1977, pp. 1–18.
You are interested in nutrition in infants, pregnant women, and adolescents	⇒	*The American Journal of Maternal-Child Nursing,* March/April 1977.
	⇒	Aubrey, R.N., et. al.: "Assessment of Maternal Nutrition," *Clinical Perinatology,* **2**(2):207–219 (September, 1975).

DECISION TABLE 2-1 (continued)

If . . .   Then . . .

⟹   McKigney, J., and Munro, H.N.
(eds.): *Nutrient Requirements in
Adolescence,* Cambridge, Mass., MIT
Press, 1976.

POSTTEST

1. Match the assessments in the left column with the instruments in the right column. Place the letters from the right column in the blanks in the left column.

   _____ Tests for sense of touch   a. Ophthalmoscope
   _____ Examination of ear   b. Percussion hammer
   _____ Measures blood pressure   c. Thermometer
   _____ Auscultation of heart sounds   d. Centimeter tape
   _____ Tests reflexes   e. Otoscope
   _____ Examination of eye   f. Cotton-tipped applicator
   _____ Measurement of Temperature   g. Stethoscope
   _____ Measures length   h. Sphygmomanometer

2. Give *three* reasons for performing a health assessment.

3. In relation to the physical examination portion of the health assessment, *five* major methods of examination are used. Name these.

4. Complete the following sentences with the appropriate method of examination.

   a. Using _____, the hand of the examiner may be used to examine the skin for texture, moisture, and masses.

   b. Using _____, heart sounds may be evaluated.

   c. Observation of the client is called _____.

   d. Using _____, the examiner strikes or taps various portions of the body and evaluates the sounds produced by the resulting vibration.

5. In assessing the growth and development level of a client, some of the behaviors listed below are normal. Other behaviors are an indication of delayed development. Indicate whether the behavior given is normal (*N*) or delayed (*D*) in the space provided to the left.

a. _____ A 6-month-old infant who does not lift head when lying prone.

b. _____ A 1-year-old who walks only when one hand is held by parent.

c. _____ A 4-year-old who cannot cut with scissors.

d. _____ A 2-year-old who has a vocabulary of "Mama," "Dada," and two or three other words.

e. _____ A 5-year-old who identifies four basic colors — red, yellow, blue, and green.

f. _____ An 18-year-old girl who has not reached menarche.

g. _____ A 14-year-old boy who feels somewhat shy and uneasy around members of the opposite sex.

h. _____ A 50-year-old man who is seeking first-time employment after years of beachcombing.

i. _____ A 20-year-old girl who is working her way through college by holding a part-time job.

j. _____ A 15-year-old boy who states that he keeps outgrowing his clothes and is 5 in taller than he was a year ago.

k. _____ A 2-year-old with two teeth.

l. _____ A mother who reports that Jill, aged 10, spends a great deal of time with her friend, Amy: "They are together all the time; I don't think it is good for any two children to be together so much."

m. _____ An 85-year-old client who likes to reminisce about the past more than to try new activities now.

6. Which of the following definitions *best* describes health?

a. Absence of illness or disease

b. Feeling good

c. A state of complete physical, mental, and social well-being

7. Vital signs are sometimes called *cardinal signs* and include what *four* procedures?

Write *true* or *false*. If *false*, correct the statement to make it true.

8. _____ Temperature is maintained by a balance between the production and the loss of heat.

9. _____ The medulla in the brain is the principle regulator of body temperature.

10. _____ Body heat is produced mainly by metabolic activity and exercise.

11. _____ Heat is lost primarily through radiation, convection, evaporation, and conduction.

12. _____ When blood vessels are in a state of vasodilation, heat is conserved by the body.

13. _____ A temperature of 93.4°F indicates pyrexia.

14. _____ Normal body temperature may vary in accordance with circadian rhythm throughout the day.

15. _____ The pulse is a measure of the number of times the left ventricle contracts in a minute.

16. _____ Stimulation by the parasympathetic system increases the pulse rate.

17. _____ *Respiration* is the term used to describe the act of breathing.

18. _____ An accumulation of carbon dioxide in the blood triggers the respiratory center in the brain and involuntary respiration occurs.

19. _____ An inadequate oxygen supply creates a condition known as *hypoxia*.

20. _____ Respiration is controlled by the hypothalamus.

21. _____ Pale skin is an indication of a condition known as *cyanosis*.

22. _____ The highest point of pressure exerted on the arteries by left-ventricle contraction is called the *diastolic pressure.*

23. _____ Peripheral resistance maintains blood pressure when arterioles are in a state of partial contraction.

24. _____ The greater the viscosity of the blood, the lower the blood pressure.

25. _____ A high cardiac output will be reflected in an increased blood pressure.

26. _____ Blood pressure may rise after exercise and when the client is anxious.

27. _____ Body position may alter the blood pressure reading.

28. _____ The DDST evaluates the range of accomplishment of the school-age child.

29. _____ The DDST is an IQ test.

30. _____ A child who is being given the DDST on July 17, 1979, and whose birthday is February 10, 1978, is 1 year, 5 months, and 7 days of age.

31. _____ A delay in the DDST is any item failed which is completely to the left of the child's age line.

32. _____ When a child earns a delay in the DDST, it means that a task cannot be performed which is achieved by 90 percent of the children at a younger age.

33. _____ The DDST is considered abnormal and referral is indicated if one section has one delay.

34. _____ An Apgar score of 2 would indicate a healthy, vigorous infant.

35. _____ A newborn with a low Apgar score 5 min after birth is likely to manifest neurological abnormalities at 1 year of age.

36. _____ Children tend to stay in the same growth percentile throughout development and should be referred for evaluation if a sudden shift in percentile occurs.

37. _____ Skin-fold measurements of nutritional status yield information on the amount of subcutaneous fat and the caloric status of the client.

38. What implications does the concept of symmetry have in conducting the physical assessment?

39. List at least *five* observations made in the general overview portion of the physical assessment.

40. A number of physical findings are listed below. Some are normal; others indicate a need for follow-up and possible referral. In the space provided to the left, indicate whether the finding is within normal limits (*N*), or will require follow-up and possible referral (*R*).

  a. _____ A 35-year-old woman who is 5 ft 0 in tall and weighs 130 lb.
  b. _____ A 75-year-old man with a BP of 140/80.
  c. _____ A 20-year-old coed with a BP of 120/100 mmHg.
  d. _____ A 2-year-old girl with the following vital signs: 99(R)-95-28 BP 96 systolic.
  e. _____ A newborn infant whose head circumference measures 35 cm and whose chest measures 33 cm.
  f. _____ A 16-year-old adolescent whose vital signs are 100-86-22.
  g. _____ A 92-year-old bedfast client whose vital signs are 99(R)-72-18.
  h. _____ A 20-year-old client who appears quite anxious and whose vital signs are 130/85-98.6-85 (bounding)-24.
  i. _____ A 45-year-old black male who is 3 ft 8 in and weighs 75 lb.

41. The DDST is divided into *four* main sections. Name these.

42. Name the *basic four* food groups:

43. Given the following 24-hour diet recall for a 24-year-old male, identify nutritional deficiencies using the basic four food groups as a tool for analysis of data.

Breakfast	**Lunch**	**Dinner**	**Snacks**
2 eggs	ham sandwich	meat loaf	1 snack bag of
3 strips bacon	potato chips	potatoes	potato chips
1 piece of toast	1 Coke	rolls, gravy	1 hamburger
1 cup of coffee	5 chocolate chip	iced tea	1 order of
	cookies		french fries
			2 Cokes

44. In the space provided to the right of descriptions, designate the body type being described.

a. Short, stocky _____

b. Well-developed, muscular _____

c. Musculature poorly developed _____

d. Face triangular in shape _____

e. Face ovoid in shape _____

f. Chest broad and short _____

g. Chest long and flat _____

h. Average height _____

i. Tall and willowy _____

HEALTH HISTORY AND ASSESSMENT

General Description of Client

Name of client _____

Birth date _____ Race _____ Sex _____

Height/length _____ Weight _____

(Child/infant) Head circumference _____ (Child/infant) Chest circumference _____

(Adult) Body build: Small frame _____ Medium frame _____ Large frame _____

Body type _____

TPR _____ Blood pressure: Sitting _____

Standing _____

Lying _____

Pulse pressure ____

General appearance
(Grooming, hygiene, hair color, eye color, facial expression)

Apparent age _____

Stature, posture, gait, quality of movements

Growth and developmental assessment

(Newborn) Apgar score _____

(Child, birth to age 6) Results of DDST _____

Present developmental tasks or behaviors

Nutritional status

24-hour dietary recall _____

_____

Skin-fold measurements:

Deltoid triceps _____ Subscapular _____ Upper abdomen _____

Client's description of current health status

Speech patterns
(Language spoken, use of vocabulary, flow of ideas, pace of words, tone of voice)

Odors present

Body _____

Breath _____

Personality

Mood _____

_____

Anxiety level _____

_____

Level of awareness _____

_____

Characteristic or unusual behavior _____

_____

Level of intelligence _____

_____

Attitude toward examiner _____

_____

Presence of abnormalities (describe)

Use of eyeglasses _____

Use of dentures _____

Use of crutches, prostheses, etc. _____

Presence of chronic illness for which client is being treated (describe) _____

_____

Missing or deformed limbs _____

Lesions, scars, discolorations on skin _____

Other _____

Recommendations, treatment, or disposition of abnormal findings:

Student_____

INSTRUCTOR'S GUIDE FOR EVALUATION OF STUDENT PERFOR-MANCE

For evaluation of student performance, student should have experience with an adult and a pediatric client below the age of 5.

Behaviors evaluated	Yes	No	Remarks
1. Able to identify five instruments used in physical assessment and give example of how each is used			
2. Develops an overview of an adult client			
3. Provides for privacy of client during assessment			
4. Drapes patient to avoid undue exposure during assessment			
5. Obtains height and weight and reports findings in pounds and ounces			
6. Obtains oral and axillary temperature using correct technique and equipment and reports results accurately			
7. Obtains respirations using correct technique			
8. Obtains BP using correct technique and equipment			
9. Calculates pulse pressure accurately			
10. Is able to state the normal ranges for TPR, BP in adult			
11. Selects an appropriate method for assessing nutritional status (24-hour recall, 3-day food intake, skin-fold measurement, or height-weight table comparison)			
12. Correctly identifies at least 3 developmental tasks appropriate for client			
13. Correctly identifies the client's body type			
14. Inspects client for			
a. Description of apparent health			
b. Race, sex			
c. Eye, hair, skin color			
d. Height, weight			
e. Apparent age			
f. Description of body type			
g. Symmetry, coordination, body movement, gait			
h. Respirations			

Behaviors evaluated	Yes	No	Remarks
15. Palpates			
a. Radial pulse			
b. Body temperature			
c. Brachial artery			
16. Auscultates			
a. Apical pulse			
b. Korotkoff sounds			
17. Percusses			
a. Posterior lung fields			
b. Abdomen over stomach			
c. Thigh			
(Describes difference in sound produced)			
Evaluation of pediatric client (below age 5):			
18. Cites at least three developmental tasks appropriate for child examined			
19. Conducts DDST using appropriate technique			
20. Records findings of DDST accurately			
21. Obtains head circumference using correct technique and records using centimeters			
22. Obtains chest circumference using correct technique and records in centimeters			
23. Obtains length and weight using correct technique			
24. Is able to identify growth percentile in which child belongs			
25. Obtains BP using correct equipment and technique			
26. Obtains temperature using correct route and technique			
27. Obtains pulse using correct technique			
28. Obtains respirations by correct technique			
29. Is able to state normal ranges of values for TPR, BP for pediatric client			
30. Records all findings in correct terms			
31. Is able to identify overt deviations from normal			

Comments:

Instructor _____ Date _____

MODULE 3

INTEGUMENTARY ASSESSMENT

This module will begin your study of assessment of body systems and, as such, should prove exciting. The authors wish to remind you that though physical assessment is important, careful and complete history taking for the system under study must be done to set physical findings in the appropriate context of meaning for an individual client.

Integument, simply defined, means covering and for the purpose of this module will include the skin, hair, and nails. Techniques of examination to be used in evaluation of this system will include inspection, palpation, and olfaction. Emphasis will be placed on accurate observation and recording of findings on the health history and physical forms provided. Differences in normal findings in assessment of the integument of the child and geriatric client are presented and are to be utilized in recording and evaluating the data you collect.

In format this module is similar to preceding modules. You are to complete the Pretest and pass the Posttest before proceeding to the skills laboratory for assessment of the integumentary system.

If you have difficulty in completing this module, contact your instructor.

PREREQUISITE OBJECTIVES

You should be able to:

1. Cite at least four functions of the skin.
2. Name the three main layers of skin.
3. Name the organs located in each layer of skin and describe the functions of each.
4. Label the structures, using a diagram of skin and its organs.

5. Identify the anatomical parts, using a diagram of a nail and underlying structure.
6. Describe the structure of a hair and its relationship to the hair follicle.
7. Describe the composition and function of sebum secreted by the sebaceous glands.
8. Describe the function of the sweat gland and its product, perspiration.
9. Describe the differences in sweat secreted by the eccrine sweat glands and the apocrine glands.
10. Describe the types of bacterial flora normally present on the skin.
11. State the normal pH of the skin.

TERMINAL OBJECTIVES

Upon completion of this module you are expected to be able to:

1. Define vocabulary words accompanying this module.
2. Describe techniques of examination to be used in assessment of the integumentary system.
3. List eight observations to be made in assessment of the skin.
4. List and define the five criteria used in assessing skin lesions.
5. Differentiate between primary and secondary skin lesions.
6. Identify five types of primary skin lesions.
7. Identify at least five types of secondary skin lesions.
8. Demonstrate inspection of the integumentary system.
9. Demonstrate palpation of the integumentary system.
10. Describe changes in the integumentary system that accompany biologic aging.
11. Describe the integumentary system of the newborn.
12. Describe common skin alterations during pregnancy.
13. Describe differences in skin color due to ethnic variation.
14. List at least five observations that should be made in assessment of the nails.
15. Describe the quantity and distribution of the three specialized types of hair to be found on examination.
16. List at least five observations that should be made in assessment of the hair.
17. Demonstrate evaluation for foreign bodies in the hair.
18. Describe the normal patterns of dermatoglyphics on hands and feet.
19. Demonstrate securing palm and footprint for evaluation of dermatoglyphics.
20. Given an assessment form as a guide, take a health history pertinent to the integumentary system using appropriate branching questions.
21. Given an assessment form as a guide, perform an assessment of the integumentary system on an adult or child as required by the instructor.
22. Record data on history and physical form using correct terminology.

**SUGGESTED
ACTIVITIES**

Read

Alexander, Mary, and Marie Brown: "The Skin," *Pediatric History Taking and Physical Diagnosis for Nurses,* McGraw-Hill, New York, 1979.

Bates, Barbara: "The Skin" and "Pediatric Physical Examination: The Skin," *A Guide to Physical Examination,* Lippincott, Philadelphia, 1979.

Luckmann, Joan, and Karen Sorenson: *Medical-Surgical Nursing: A Psychophysiologic Approach,* Saunders, Philadelphia, 1974, pp. 1251-1254, 1260 (pediculosis).

Malasanos, Lois, et al.: "Assessment of the Skin," "Assessment of the Pediatric Client: Skin," and "Assessment of the Geriatric Client: Skin," *Health Assessment,* Mosby, St. Louis, 1977.

Roach, Lora: "Color Changes in Dark Skins," *Nursing '77,* 48-51 (January, 1977), or *Nursing '72,* 19-22 (November, 1972).

Saxon, Sue V., and Mary Jean Etten: "The Integument," *Physical Change and Aging: A Guide for the Helping Professions,* The Tiresias Press, New York, 1978.

Ziegel, Erna, and Mecca Cranley: "Maternal Physiologic Changes During Pregnancy—Skin," *Obstetric Nursing,* Macmillan, New York, 1978.

OR

Reeder, Sharon R., et al.: "Normal Pregnancy—Changes in Various Systems, Skin," *Maternity Nursing,* Lippincott, Philadelphia, 1976.

View

Physical Assessment: The Skin and Extremities, Trainex program 451.

Physical Examination of the School Aged Child: The Integumentary System, Trainex program 498.

Biologic Changes of Aging: Physical Appearance and the Special Senses, frames 15 to 29, Trainex program 453.

Equipment

magnifying glass

centimeter ruler

fine-tooth comb

fingerprinting pad and paper

Wood's lamp (for advanced student)

PRETEST

1. List at least *four* functions of the skin.

_____

_____

_____

_____

2. Label the *three* major layers of skin on Fig. 3-1.

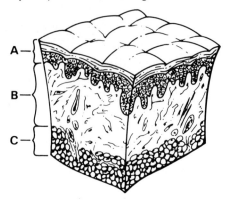

Figure 3-1

3. On Fig. 3-2, label the structures indicated.

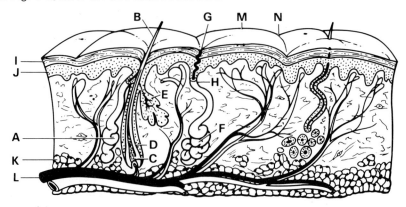

Figure 3-2

4. Label the parts of Fig. 3-3 as indicated.

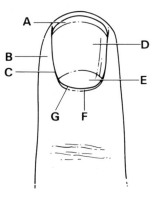

Figure 3-3

Write *true* or *false.* If *false,* correct the statement to make it true.

5. _____ The skin comprises 15 percent of the body weight.

6. _____ The epidermis is uniformly thin over most of the body and measures 1.5 to 4 mm.

7. _____ Two major types of cells can be located in the epidermis — melanocytes and keratinocytes.

8. _____ The epidermis is completely replaced about every three months by cell mitosis and removal of dead cells.

9. _____ Flexibility or elasticity of the skin is dependent on a desirable water content of the outer layer.

10. _____ Differences in the amount of pigment among ethnic groups result from the differences in the rate and quality of production of melanin.

11. _____ The chief components of sweat are sodium, chloride, calcium, nitrates, and carbonates.

12. _____ Unless fever is present, eccrine glands in the hands and palms produce sweat only upon emotional stimulation.

13. _____ Apocrine glands respond to emotional stimulation and produce a milky and distinctly alkaline perspiration.

14. _____ Body odor is caused by bacterial decomposition of the products of the eccrine sweat glands.

15. _____ Sebum, secreted by the arrectores pilorum, is produced by a degeneration of the hair follicle plus an accumulation of fat.

16. _____ The activity of the sebaceous glands is stimulated by estrogen.

17. _____ Anagen, catagen, and telogen are the cyclic changes in hair development.

18. _____ A major function of the nail is to protect the delicate nerve endings which produce the sense of touch.

19. _____ The major function of the dermis is to provide protection for the cutaneous adipose tissue.

20. _____ Collagen forms the greatest part of the substance of the dermis.

21. _____ Sensory fibers form a complex dermal network.

22. _____ Group B hemalytic streptococci are among the normal bacterial flora of human skin.

23. _____ The normal pH of the skin (7.5 to 8.6) retards the growth of pathogens on the skin.

Three major types of hair are listed. Match each of these with the appropriate description from the column at the right.

24. _____ Vellus   a. Fine nonpigmented hair that covers parts of the body

25. _____ Terminal hair   b. Fine hair that covers the body during fetal life and disappears shortly after birth

26. _____ Lanugo   c. Coarse, long, pigmented hair that covers all normally hairy parts of the body

VOCABULARY

Descriptive terminology

acne vulgaris	hirsutism	perspiration
alopecia	hyperpigmentation	physiologic jaundice
angioma	hypopigmentation	pilosebaceous unit
apocrine glands	integument	plaque
bullae	jaundice	pustule
carbuncle	keloid	rash
carotenemia	keratin	reticular
chloasma	keratosis	scale
collagen	lanugo	seborrhea
crepitus	lunula	Simian line or crease
crust	lichenification	striae
cyanosis	linea alba	striae albicantes
cysts	linea nigra	striae gravidarum
decubitus ulcer	maceration	sweat
dermatoglyphics	macule	telangiectasia
dermatology	melanin	tenting
desquamation	milia	triradii
ecchymoses	Mongolian spots	tumor
eccrine glands	morphology	turgor
eczema	nevus	ulcer
eponychium	nevus flammeus	varicosity
erosion	(port-wine stain)	vernix caseosa
erythema	nodule	vesicle
excoriation	pallor	vitiligo
fissure	papule	wheal
harlequin sign	pediculosis	xanthoma
hemangioma	petechiae	

Diagnostic terminology (for the advanced student)

athlete's foot	pityriasis rosea
atopic dermatitis	psoriasis
basal-cell carcinoma	rubella
café au lait spot	rubeola
decubitus ulcers	scarlatina
dermatosis papulosa nigra	scabies
erythema multiforme	seborrheic dermatitis
erythema toxicum neonatorum	seborrheic keratosis
furuncle	senile keratosis
herpes simplex	squamous cell carcinoma
herpes zoster	tinea capitis
impetigo contagiosa	tinea corporis
intertrigo	tinea versicolor
malignant melanoma	urticaria
paronychia	varicella

DECISION TABLE 3-1

If . . .		Then . . .
You need to review anatomy and physiology of the integument	⟹	Read the chapter concerning the skin or integument in your anatomy and physiology textbook.
	⟹	Luckmann, Joan, and Karen Sorenson: *Medical-Surgical Nursing: A Psychophysiologic Approach,* Saunders, Philadelphia, 1974, pp. 1249-1251.
You would like pictorial assistance in visualizing material	⟹	Abbott Laboratories, *Common Skin Diseases, an Atlas,* North Chicago, Ill.
	⟹	Mead Johnson and Company, *No. 1: The Skin* and *No. 4: Birthmarks,* Evansville, Ind., 1972 (information about infants).
Additional or alternate audiovisual media	⟹	*Integument,* Blue-Hill Educational Systems videotape, 60 min.
You would like further instruction on performing an assessment of the integumentary system	⟹	Roach, Lora B.: "Skin Changes: The Subtle and Obvious," *Assessing Vital Functions Accurately,* Nursing '77 Books—Intermed Communications, 1977, pp. 33-46.
You don't want to miss a brief but excellent article on black skin (this article includes some descriptive photographs)	⟹	Kenny, John A.: "Skin Problems of Blacks," *Journal of the American Medical Association,* **236**(3): 301-303 (July 19, 1976).
You wish further discussion and some additional photographs aiding in assessment of dermatological conditions in blacks	⟹	Galles, Mary L.: "Identifying Dermatological Conditions in Blacks," *Journal of Emergency Nursing,* **4**(6):56-62 (November-December, 1978).
You would like an additional pediatric reference	⟹	Barness, Lewis: *Manual of Pediatric Diagnosis,* Year Book, Chicago, 1972, pp. 19-38.
	⟹	Brown, Marie, and Mary Alexander: "Physical Examination: Part 3, Examining the Skin," *Nursing '73,* 39-43 September, 1973)
	⟹	Chinn, Peggy L., and Cynthia Leitch: *Child Health Maintenance: A Guide to Clinical Assessment,* Mosby, St. Louis, 1979, pp. 21-22, 24, 95-97.
You need a reference on the black child	⟹	McLaughtin, Clara: *Black Parents Handbook,* Harcourt Brace Jovanovich, New York, 1976, pp. 82-86.

DECISION TABLE 3-1 (continued)

If . . .

You are interested in assessment of the skin in the newborn ⟹ Korones, Sheldon R.: *High Risk Newborn Infants,* Mosby, St. Louis, 1976, pp. 104-107.

You would like additional geriatric references ⟹ Burnside, Irene Mortonson: *Nursing and the Aged,* McGraw-Hill, New York, 1976, pp. 83-84, 91.

⟹ Caird, F. I., and T. G. Judge: *Assessment of the Elderly,* Pitman, Calif., pp. 22-24.

⟹ Hayter, Jean: "Biologic Changes of Aging," *Nursing Forum,* **13**(3):289-308 (1974).

This geriatric reference includes some fine photographs of common skin changes ⟹ Uhler, Diana M.: "Common Skin Changes in the Elderly," *American Journal of Nursing,* **78**(8):1342-1344 (August, 1978).

For an overview of skin changes in the pregnant client ⟹ Kahn, G.: "Skin Problems in Pregnancy: Skin Changes Normal in Pregnancy," *Consultant,* 201 (November, 1976).

You would like additional information on dermatoglyphics ⟹ Holt, Sara B.: "Dermatoglyphics," *Nursing Mirror,* 16-19 (July 20, 1973).

You love different approaches to familiar subject and have some time to read just for fun ⟹ Selzer, Richard: *Mortal Lessons: Notes on the Art of Surgery,* Simon & Schuster, New York, 1976, pp. 105-115.

You like things explained in a way you are sure to understand and enjoy and you still have some free time, or you are planning an educational program for elementary school children ⟹ Allison, Linda: "Skin, the Bag You Live In," *Blood and Guts,* Little, Brown, Boston, 1976, pp. 11-20.

For the more advanced student

You are seeking a good overview of common skin disorders and their management ⟹ Luckmann, Joan, and Karen Sorenson: *Medical-Surgical Nursing: A Psychophysiologic Approach,* Saunders, Philadelphia, 1974, pp. 1254-1276.

Good overview of common clinical syndromes with black and white photographs of these disorders is desired ⟹ Delp, Mahlon, and Robert T. Manning: *Major's Physical Diagnosis,* Saunders, Philadelphia, 1975, pp. 88-117.

You want good photographs with discussion of disorders commonly seen in practice ⟹ Derbes, Vincent J.: "Rashes: Recognition and Management," *Nursing '78,* 54-59 (March, 1978).

DECISION TABLE 3-1 (continued)

If . . .		Then . . .
Infants and children are your special area of interest and you like programmed materials, this is an excellent source for information on pediatric assessment	⟹	Cohen, Stephen, and Geraldine Glass: "Skin Rashes in Infants and Children," *American Journal of Nursing,* 1043-1069 (June, 1978) (a programmed unit).
You need an introduction to skin rashes and foreign bodies commonly found in school children and their management (includes color photos)	⟹	Rice, Alice K.: "Common Skin Infections in School Children," *American Journal of Nursing,* 1905-1910 (November, 1973).
You would like an introduction to rashes caused by drugs	⟹	Derbes, Vincent: "Rashes—Recognition and Management," *Nursing '73,* 44-49 (March, 1973).
You would like a more in-depth look at assessment of skin color and temperature and their significance (this may prove particularly helpful if you will work in intensive-care areas or with long-term chronic illnesses)	⟹	Roberts, Sharon L.: "Skin Assessment for Color and Temperature," *American Journal of Nursing,* 610-613 (April, 1975).
You need an introduction to evaluation of the skin for precancerous and cancerous lesions (illustrations included)	⟹	Clark, Wallace, et al.: "Skin Cancer: Early Detection Is the Key to Survival," *Nursing Update,* 3-8 (June, 1975).

POSTTEST

1. Name the three techniques of assessment used in evaluation of the integumentary system.

Write *true* or *false.* If *false,* correct the statement to make it true.

2. _____ The client's emotional state may affect skin color.

3. _____ Recent cigarette smoking may affect the color of the nail beds.

4. _____ It is important to remove dirt and soil before inspecting the integument, as its presence may mask clinically significant lesions.

5. _____ Artificial lighting is preferred when performing an examination of the integument.

6. _____ The examiner palpates for skin temperature using the fingertips or the palm of the hand.

7. _____ Moisture is determined by palpation of the palms, upper lip, and forehead.

8. _____ Increased levels of carotenoid pigment or carotenemia causes the sclera to turn yellow.

9. _____ In examining color changes in dark-skinned individuals, the most accurate assessment can be obtained from inspection of the sclera, conjunctiva, nail beds, tongue, and buccal mucosa.

10. _____ Dehydration may be determined by pressing fingers firmly against the skin. Dehydration is present if an impression remains when the fingers are removed.

11. _____ Dehydration is a serious finding in any age group. For infants, it is life-threatening and they must be referred to the physician immediately.

12. _____ *Fair, tan, dark, olive, cyanotic, jaundiced* are terms used to describe changes in moles.

13. _____ *Foul, musky, strong, fruity, pungent* are terms used to describe data obtained by olfaction.

14. _____ Secondary lesions occur when there are evolutionary changes in primary lesions or when trauma has occurred.

15. _____ In the geriatric client, the skin loses its elasticity due to an increase in the production of collagen.

16. Accurate description of lesions is based upon *five* criteria. Name these.

_____

_____

_____

_____

_____

17. Classify the following skin lesions as *primary* or *secondary.*

crust _____   scar_____

macule _____   tumor _____

plaque_____   ulcer _____

nodule_____   bulla _____

cyst_____   fissure_____

18. Match the descriptions of lesions in the left column with the names of lesions in the right column.

_____ Scratch or superficial injury	1. Macule
_____ A raised lesion containing fluid and greater than 0.5 cm	2. Nodule
	3. Tumor
_____ A confluence of papules	4. Plaque
_____ Irregular, edematous lesion	5. Wheal or hive
_____ Purple-red hemorrhagic spots	6. Vesicle
_____ Discolored spot or patch that is seen and not felt	7. Bulla
	8. Excoriation
_____ Solid lesion exceeding 1 cm in diameter	9. Petechiae
_____ Blue-black irregular bruises	10. Ecchymosis
_____ Raised lesion containing clear fluid that measures less than 0.5 cm	
_____ A solid lesion measuring between 0.5 and 1 cm	

19. Identify the lesions shown in Fig. 3-4.

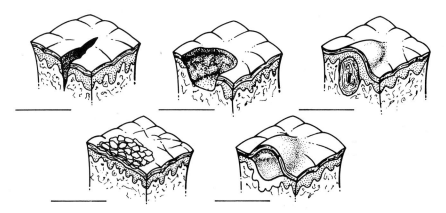

Figure 3-4

20. Identify the dermatoglyphics shown on the hand in Fig. 3-5.

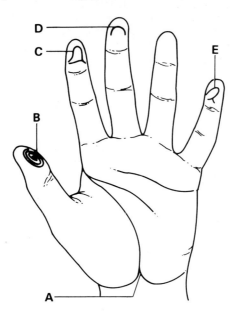

Figure 3-5

The following conditions should be marked *normal* or *abnormal*. *Abnormal* conditions are those for which you would perform a further work-up or refer to the physician.

21. _____ Examination of an infant reveals tufts of hair over the sacrum.

22. _____ Examination of infant (6 hours old) reveals cyanosis of the hands and feet— the examiner notes that the feet are darker than the hands.

23. _____ Examination of a newborn reveals small yellow fat plaques across the nose.

24. _____ Examination of a Spanish-American infant discloses two half-dollar-size bluish discolorations of the skin over the coccygeal area.

25. _____ Examination of newborn reveals an abrupt line of demarcation at the midline with one side of the body being red and the other pale.

26. _____ Examination of gums of a Negro male reveals bluish pigmentation distributed in splotches.

27. _____ Dark-skinned person whose color could best be described as *ash* or *gray*.

28. _____ Yellowish tint of the palate in a dark-skinned individual.

29. _____ Presence of hair in axilla and pubic area of a 7-year-old girl.

30. _____

Figure 3-6

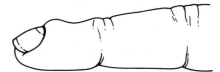

31. _____

Figure 3-7

32. _____

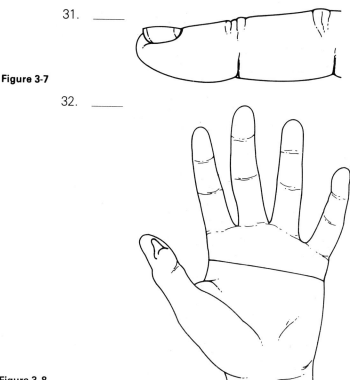

Figure 3-8

33. _____ A number of cherry angiomas located on the trunk of a 75-year-old white female.

34. _____ Small white foreign bodies in the hair, extremely difficult to remove even with a fine-tooth comb.

35. _____ Patches of absence of color on the arms and face of a Spanish-American female.

36. _____ A mole of variegated color — red, blue, and white — on the forearm of a farmer.

37. _____ During a routine GYN examination, hair is noted within the labia of a 26-year-old Spanish-American female.

38. _____ Gray hair of a 76-year-old client.

39. _____ Broad flat nose of a Negro client.

40. _____ Hairline beginning in midforehead of a Spanish-American infant.

41. _____ Multiple papules following the pattern of the beard in a black male.

42. _____ Loss of hair around scalp margins in a 7-year-old black female client.

43. _____ Wrinkling of skin of a 73-year-old Caucasian female.

44. _____ Dry, scaly skin over the extremities of an 86-year-old female.

45. _____ Red blotchy areas on the forearms of a 90-year-old Caucasian male.

46. Match the following terms and definitions:

_____ striae gravidarum

_____ striae albicantes

_____ linea nigra

_____ linea alba

_____ chloasma

1. Silver striations of the abdomen resulting from previous pregnancies
2. A white line dividing the pregnant abdomen longitudinally
3. Pinkish and/or bluish striations of the abdomen of a pregnant woman
4. The mask of pregnancy
5. A progressive form of linea alba; a dark line dividing the pregnant abdomen longitudinally

HEALTH HISTORY AND ASSESSMENT

Adult Health History: Integumentary System

If the answer is yes, place a check (✓) at the left and provide further information in the Remarks column.

Skin   Remarks

Normal color _____

Ethnic group _____

Have you had or do you now have:

_____ Medication for skin diseases?

_____ Medications which caused your skin to break out?

_____ Any skin diseases?

_____ Changes in color of skin?

_____ Changes in temperature?

_____ Dryness?

_____ Oiliness?

_____ Excessive moisture?

_____ Itching?

_____ Rashes?

_____ Tenderness?

_____ Any unusual discoloration or pigmentation of skin?

_____ Changes in warts or moles?

_____ Allergies or hives?

_____ Allergic response to soap or bubble bath?

_____ Allergic response to deodorants, feminine hygiene deodorant sprays, perfumes, etc.?

_____ Swelling, lump, or growth?

_____ Changes in body odor?

_____ Sensitivity to sun?

_____ Birthmarks?

_____ Delayed healing of wounds?

_____ Bruising that occurs easily?

_____ Bleeding that occurs easily?

_____ Athlete's foot or skin fungus?

_____ Skin tests; if yes, what type?

_____

Result?_____

_____ Recent injury to skin?

_____ Exposure to chemicals?

_____ Exposure to x-ray?

_____ Subject to boils?

_____ Subject to fever blisters?

_____ Sensitive to insect bites (bee stings, mosquito bites)?

_____ Any systemic disease for which you are receiving treatment? If so, explain _____

_____

_____ Keloid formation?

_____ Frequency of shaving? _____

Areas shaved?_____

Shaving preparation used? _____

_____

Type of razor used? _____

Hair

Usual color_____

_____ Have you used dyes, hair straighteners, electrical appliances such as curling irons, hot rollers?

Have you had or do you now have:

_____ Disease of the hair or scalp?

_____ Change in amount or distribution of body hair?

_____ Change in color of hair without use of dyes, etc.?

_____ Hair loss?

_____ Brittleness or breaking?

_____ Dryness?

_____ Oiliness?

_____ Itching of scalp?

_____ Problems with dandruff or scaling of scalp?

_____ Change in odor of hair?

_____ Hair pulling or twisting?

_____ Baldness?

_____ Loss of pubic or axillary hair?

_____ Foreign bodies in hair (example: pediculosis)?

_____ Brands of shampoo and rinses

used?_____

_____ Frequency of shampooing?

_____ Use of medication on hair or scalp?

_____ Presently taking any medication? If so, please list:

_____

_____

Nails

_____ Disease of the nails?

_____ Nail biting?

_____ Brittleness?

_____ Changes in color?

_____ Loss or absence of nail?

_____ Frequent hangnail?

_____ Loose or floating nail?

_____ Ridging or pitting?

_____ Pain?

_____ Growths under nail?

_____ Frequent contact with chemicals?

_____ Extended immersion in water?

_____ Redness or swelling around nail?

_____ Traumatic injury to nail?

_____ Nutritional disease?

_____ Type of nail polish used?

_____ Artificial-nail use?

Pediatric Adaptation History

Infant

Presenting part during delivery? _____

_____ Use of forceps for delivery?

Length of labor? _____

_____ Difficult labor?

Older infant and child

_____ Frequent diaper rash?

_____ Difficulty with cradle cap?

_____ Frequent falls?

_____ Frequent corporal punishment required?

_____ Allergic skin responses after introduction of new foods?

_____ Allergic responses following use of soap, shampoo, or bubble bath?

Adolescent

_____ Blackheads?

_____ Pimples?

_____ Excessive oiliness?

_____ Adverse skin response to consumption of special foods (french fries, etc.)

Describe type of skin- and hair-care products used: _____

_____

Describe skin- and hair-care routine: _____

_____

_____ Presently seeing physician for skin-care treatment?

Geriatric Adaptations— History

_____ Increase in dryness or scaliness of skin?

_____ Itching?

_____ Bruise easily? Any discolored areas?

Remarks

_____ Raised, black, warty areas on body?

_____ Pressure areas? Soreness? Redness?

Ethnic Adaptations— History

Black client

_____ History of sickle cell anemia?

_____ Problems with skin ulcerations?

Adult Physical Assessment— Integumentary System

Check (✔) if normal, *NE* if not examined, and *X* if abnormal. Describe abnormal findings.

Skin   Description

Color_____

Temperature _____

Texture _____

_____ No varicosities, distended veins, or telangiectasis

_____ No scars or distinguishing marks

_____ No striae

_____ No lesions

_____ No edema

_____ Turgor good

_____ No unusual odors

_____ No excessive dryness or oiliness (the skin of a black client will normally be drier than that of a Caucasian client)

_____ No reddened areas or pressure sores

_____ No crepitus

_____ No pain on palpation

_____ No bruises or petechiae

_____ Evidence of good hygiene present

_____ No track marks or scars.

Hair

Color_____

Texture _____

Amount_____

Curled or straight _____

_____ Color distributed evenly

_____ No alopecia

_____ No evidence of traumatic
marginal alopecia (from tight
braids, hot curlers, "corn-
rowing")

_____ No dandruff or scaling of scalp

_____ No foreign bodies

_____ No lesions on scalp

_____ Hair distributed evenly
bilaterally

_____ No hirsutism

_____ No unusual odors

_____ Evidence of good hygiene
present

_____ No excessive oiliness or
dryness (hair of a black client
will normally be dryer than that
of Caucasian client)

_____ No brittleness or broken ends

_____ No abnormal distribution or
pattern of body hair

_____ Hairline on scalp begins well
above eyebrows except in
clients of Spanish-American
descent, where it may begin in
midforehead

Nails

Color of nail plate _____

_____ Angle of nail at base 160°

_____ Consistency hard

_____ Capillary return good

_____ All nails present

_____ Nail plate semitransparent, convex, rectangular (longer than wide)

_____ White, crescent-shaped lunula

_____ Nail plate smooth

_____ Skin surrounding nail plate pink and free from irritation

_____ Free edge intact

_____ No thickening of nail plate

_____ No alteration in angle between nail and finger

_____ No movement of nail plate when pressed

_____ No clubbing

Dermatoglyphics

Palm:

_____ Displays triradius at wrist

_____ 7 to 8 fingertips show ulnar loops

_____ 1 to 3 fingertips show whorls

_____ One or no arches present

_____ No simian crease

Sole:

_____ Whorls or loops in hallucal (ball) area

Treatment, disposition, and recommendations regarding abnormal findings

(Example: reevaluate in one week, refer to physician, etc.)

Pediatric Adaptations— Physical

Neonate

_____ Vernix caseosa present

_____ Scaliness and desquamation in newborns within normal limits

_____ Physiological jaundice (appears past 24 hours of life and clears before seventh day)

Description

_____ Acrocyanosis less marked
in hands than in feet

_____ Telangiectatic nevi (stork bite)

Size and location: _____

_____

_____ Xanthomas may be present

_____ Milia

_____ No erythema toxicum
neonatorum past first 3 days
of life

_____ Harlequin sign

_____ Edema not present after
second or third day

_____ Lanugo covers entire body

_____ Mongolian spots present only if
infant is black, Spanish-
American, Indian, or Oriental

_____ Birthmarks (describe)_____

_____

_____ Absence of depressed fontanels

_____ Turgor good

Infant/child

_____ No bruises or lesions in unusual
or unlikely places*

_____ Hair and scalp free of foreign
bodies

**Geriatric
Adaptations—
Physical**

Description

_____ Dry, wrinkled skin

_____ Diminished subcutaneous fat

_____ Scaly skin

_____ Thinning of skin

_____ Brown pigmented spots on
backs of hands, wrists, face

_____ Red blotches on skin surfaces

*Great care must be taken in the observation and assessment of the location of bruises and other lesions on children. If the parent's story concerning the acquisition of such bruises and lesions does not seem to match the physical findings, then the possibility of child abuse must be considered.

_____ Thinning of hair

_____ Graying of hair

_____ Nails tough and brittle

_____ No lesions with crusts or scales

_____ No keratosis

_____ No redness or tissue breakdown over pressure areas

_____ No ulceration or discoloration of legs

Ethnic Adaptations— Physical

Black, Oriental, American-Indian babies

_____ Mongolian spots
Size and location: _____

Black client

_____ Freckling pigmentation of buccal cavity

_____ Bluish pigmentation on gums

_____ Hypo- or hyperpigmented areas

Describe: _____

_____ Keloids

Describe: _____

_____ Ulcers on legs around ankles (round ulcers with a grayish base and undermined edges are indicative of sickle cell anemia)

_____ (Children between 2 and 8) Edema of hands and feet accompanied by pain over metacarpals and phalanges (suspect sickle cell anemia)

Description

Student_____

INSTRUCTOR'S GUIDE FOR EVALUATION OF STUDENT PERFOR-MANCE	Behaviors evaluated	Yes	No	Remarks
	1. Takes appropriate history of integumentary system*			
	2. Asks appropriate branching questions*			
	3. Assembles equipment needed for assessment			
	4. Washes hands			
	5. Explains examination to client			
	6. Has client remove lipstick, nail polish, hair pieces, etc.			
	7. Provides adequate lighting (daylight, if possible)			
	8. Drapes and gowns to reduce unnecessary exposure			
	9. Inspects skin surfaces			
	10. Palpates skin surfaces to evaluate lesions, consistency, shadows			
	11. Inspects sclera and mucous membranes as part of color determination			
	12. Palpates for skin temperature contralaterally using back of fingers			
	13. Palpates with fingertips for edema by creating pressure over ankles, tibia, and sacrum			
	14. Palpates for skin turgor by pinching skin fold to test for tenting			
	15. Inspects nails			
	16. Palpates nails			
	17. Applies blanching test to nails			
	18. Inspects hair			
	19. Inspects scalp			
	20. Palpates scalp			
	21. If foreign bodies are present in hair, uses fine-tooth comb in assessing for nits; uses Wood's light for tinea capitis and other fungal infections			
	22. (Optional) Evaluates for dermatoglyphics using finger and palm prints			

*These items may be evaluated on the basis of previously submitted history.

Behaviors evaluated	Yes	No	Remarks
23. Records findings using appropriate terminology*			
24. If lesions present, data recorded concerning them must include morphology, color, configuration, distribution, and size (reported in centimeters).†			

*These items may be evaluated on basis of previously submitted history.
†This item *must* be performed correctly.

Instructor _____ Date _____

MODULE 4

ASSESSMENT OF THE HEAD AND NECK, PART 1 (EYE)

This instructional module is designed as a guide to assist you in learning a thorough and systematic approach to assessment of the eye, including visual activity, and the use of the ophthalmoscope. The use of a good instrument and repeated practice is necessary for gaining skill in performing an accurate assessment of the internal eye.

For instructor convenience, the Posttest and instructor's evaluation guide pertaining to the internal eye are separate from the other materials, for use with the advanced student.

Adaptations for assessing the infant, child, and geriatric client are included. Some ethnic variations are also included. The Pretest is to test your knowledge of anatomy and physiology of the eye, including the cranial nerves that control this organ. You are to complete this module and pass the Posttest before the scheduled laboratory period for assessment of the head and neck, part 1.

If you have difficulty in completing this module, contact your instructor.

PREREQUISITE OBJECTIVES

You should be able to:

1. Label the anatomical structures of the external eye on a diagram or model of the eye.
2. Label the anatomical structures of the internal eye on a diagram or model of the eye.
3. Describe the normal position of the eyelids.
4. Describe the physiology of vision.
5. List the names and functions of the cranial nerves that control the eye.

TERMINAL OBJECTIVES

Upon completion of this module you are expected to be able to:

1. Define the vocabulary words accompanying this module.
2. Take a complete health history pertinent to eyes, using appropriate branching questions.
3. Describe the normal color of the sclera and conjunctiva.
4. Describe normal ethnic variations in the color of the sclera of dark-skinned persons.
5. List five characteristics of the external eye that should be assessed.
6. Demonstrate the test for lid lag.
7. Administer a test for visual acuity, using the Snellen alphabet chart or Snellen E chart.
8. Interpret visual-acuity chart readings.
9. Demonstrate the procedure for testing direct and consensual reaction of pupils to light.
10. Demonstrate the procedure for testing pupillary reaction to accommodation.
11. Describe a method of assessing gross visual acuity in an infant, a preschool child, and an adult.
12. Demonstrate the procedure for assessing extraocular movements.
13. Perform Hirschberg's corneal light reflex test and interpret the findings.
14. Perform the cover test for tropia and interpret the findings.
15. Describe the landmarks that should be assessed when doing an opthalmoscopic examination.
16. Demonstrate the proper use of the ophthalmoscope.
17. Describe the normal characteristics of the disk, the physiologic cup, and the macula.
18. Describe the normal appearance of the retinal blood vessels.
19. Name two differences in the appearance of the retinal arterioles and venules.
20. Describe two abnormalities of the background of the fundus and macula.
21. Describe normal ethnic variations in the appearance of the fundus of a dark-skinned person.
22. List five abnormalities of the internal eye that require referral.
23. Perform a complete assessment of eyes, using an assessment form as a guide.
24. Describe the anatomical differences of the structures of the eye among the newborn, child, and adult that will be of significance to the examiner.
25. Describe the visual changes that can occur with aging.
26. Describe variations in characteristics of the eyes and eyelids among ethnic groups.
27. Record the data obtained from the health assessment using correct medical terminology.

SUGGESTED ACTIVITIES

Read

Alexander, Mary, and Marie Brown: "Eyes," *Pediatric History Taking and Physical Diagnosis for Nurses,* McGraw-Hill, New York, 1979.

Bates, Barbara: "The Eye" and "Pediatric Physical Examination: The Eye," *Guide to Physical Examination,* Lippincott, Philadelphia, 1979.

OR

Malasanos, Lois, et al.: "The Eye" and "Assessment of the Pediatric Client: The Eye," *Health Assessment,* Mosby, St. Louis, 1977.

Mead Johnson and Company, *The Eyes* (the newborn infant's eyes), Evansville, Ill.

Saxon, Sue V., and Mary Jean Etten: "The Sensory Systems: Vision," *Physical Change and Aging,* The Tiresias Press, New York, 1978.

View

Assessing the Function of the Eye, Concept Media, video cassette, 28 min.
Examining the Internal Eye, Concept Media, video cassette, 25 min.
Bates, Barbara, *Examination of the Head and Neck,* Lippincott, video cassette, 13 min. (eye examination).

Equipment

    penlight

    ophthalmoscope

    cotton-tipped applicator

    Snellen alphabet chart

    card for eye cover

    ophthalmic mannequin (optional)

For pediatric exam

    Denver eye screening test

    Snellen E chart (illiterate E)

PRETEST   With books closed, test your knowledge of anatomy and physiology of the eye.

1. Using Fig. 4-1, label the following:
   a. iris
   b. pupil
   c. limbus
   d. medial canthus
   e. lateral canthus
   f. bulbar conjunctiva
   g. lacrimal gland
   h. lacrimal sac

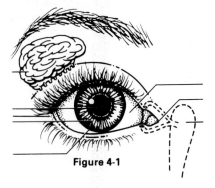

Figure 4-1

2. Using Fig. 4-2, label the following:
   a. cornea
   b. pupil
   c. iris
   d. lens
   e. fovea centralis
   f. optic nerve
   g. physiologic cup in optic disk
   h. retina
   i. choroid
   j. vitreous body
   k. anterior chamber

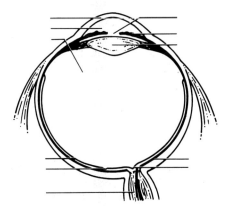

Figure 4-2

3. Match the following cranial nerve (N.) numbers with the appropriate *name* and *function.* (Include all appropriate functions that affect the eyes and vision.)

Name	Function	Name	Function
II ____	____	a. Abducens	1. Vision
III ____	____	b. Oculomotor	2. Lateral eye movement
IV ____	____	c. Optic	3. Downward, medial eye movement
V ____	____	d. Trigeminal	
VI ____	____	e. Trochlear	4. Upward, downward, medial eye movements (most of the extraocular eye movements)
			5. Elevation of upper eyelid
			6. Constriction of pupils
			7. Corneal reflex

VOCABULARY

Descriptive terminology

accommodation	hypertelorism
bulbar conjunctiva	hypotelorism
colobma	limbus
concave	macula lutea
conjunctivitis	mydriasis
consensual response	OD
convergence	OS
convex	palpebra
diopter	palpebral conjunctiva
fovea centralis	papilledema
Hirschberg's corneal light reflex test	PERRLA

Diagnostic terminology

amblyopia	chalazion	exophthalmos	nystagmus
arcus senilis	diplopia	glaucoma	presbyopia
astigmatism	ectropion	hordeolum	pterygium
Bitot's spots	entropion	hyperopia	ptosis
Brushfield's spots	esotropia	lid lag	strabismus
cataract	exotropia	myopia	tropia

DECISION TABLE 4-1

If . . .		Then . . .
You prefer programmed instruction	⟹	Mechner, Frances: "Patient Assessment: Examination of the Eye," *American Journal of Nursing* (November, 1974, and January, 1975) (well illustrated with color photographs of eye pathology).
You want thorough coverage of the opthalmoscopic examination	⟹	Prior, John A., and Jack Silberstein: *Physical Diagnosis,* Mosby, St. Louis, 1973.
You could profit from color photographs of retinal pathology	⟹	Abbott Laboratories: *Atlas of Some Pathological Conditions of the Eye, Ear, Throat,* North Chicago, Ill., pp. 6–16.
You need help with history taking and suggestions for physical examination for various eye symptoms	⟹	Wasson, John, et al.: *Common Symptom Guide,* McGraw-Hill, New York, 1975 (double vision, eye problems).

DECISION TABLE 4-1 (Continued)

If . . .		Then . . .
You need more information on testing for strabismus	⟹	Hiles, David: "Strabismus," *American Journal of Nursing*, 1082–1089 (June, 1974) (well illustrated).
	⟹	Chinn, Peggy L., and Cynthia J. Leitch: *Child Health Maintenance: A Guide to Clinical Assessment,* Mosby, St. Louis, 2d. ed., 1979. pp. 30–32, 52, 66–70.
You desire additional or alternate media	⟹	*Pediatric Physical Assessment—The Eye,* Blue-Hill Educational Systems videotape, 54 min.
	⟹	*Physical Assessment Examination—Eyes,* Blue-Hill Educational Systems videotape, 45 min.

POSTTEST

1. Interpret the meaning of a visual-acuity test result of 20/50.

   _____

2. In order to test for consensual pupil reaction to light, you would:

   _____

3. In order to test for a full range of extraocular movements, you would:

   _____

4. The cranial nerves that control extraocular movement of the eyes are:
   a. II, III, IV
   b. III, IV, VI
   c. IV, V, VI
   d. III, IV, V
5. Briefly describe Hirschberg's test for uncoordinated extraocular movements (strabismus).

   _____

   _____

6. The initials *PERRLA* are frequently used to describe the eyes. What do the letters stand for?

   P _____   R _____

   E _____   L _____

   R _____   A _____

7. Entropion is a common finding in which race or ethnic group?
   a. Caucasian
   b. Black
   c. Mexican-American
   d. American Indian
   e. Oriental

8. List *two* important findings to notice in evaluating the palpebral conjunctiva.

9. The color of the iris at birth in the white infant is usually _____ , and in the dark-skinned infant is usually _____ .

Match:

10. _____ amblyopia

11. _____ presbyopia

12. _____ exotropia

13. _____ myopia

14. _____ hyperopia

15. _____ ectropion

   a. An inward deviation of the eye
   b. An outward deviation of the eye
   c. An upward deviation of the eye
   d. Visual reduction in an anatomically normal eye
   e. A physiologic change in the eye that occurs with middle age and involves loss of accommodation
   f. Nearsightedness: light rays come to focus in front of the retina
   g. Farsightedness: light rays come to focus behind the retina
   h. A turning inward of margins of lids
   i. A turning outward of margins of lids

16. List *three* causes of a decrease in visual acuity due to the aging process.

Write *true* or *false*. If *false,* correct the statement to make it true.

17. _____ Epicanthal folds of the upper eyelids are common in both Caucasian and Oriental newborns.

18. _____ Brushfield's spots appearing in the iris of the newborn may represent an abnormal finding.

19. _____ Strabismus is a common finding in the newborn.

20. _____ Nystagmus in the newborn is abnormal and should be referred.

21. _____ Lid lag, or setting-sun sign, is frequently indicative of an abnormality.

22. _____ The doll's eye phenomenon is a normal finding in newborns.

23. _____ Ectropion and entropion are common findings in the elderly.

24. _____ Arcus senilis is a condition which should be referred.

25. _____ The corneal reflex is reduced in the elderly.

26. _____ If the infant does not blink and dorsiflex its head in response to presentation of a bright light, the examiner would note an abnormality in the Remarks column of the examining tool.

27. _____ Amblyopia is the most prevalent eye disorder in children, and treatment will be greatly reduced in effectiveness if began after age 6.

28. _____ In the normal Hirschberg's test, the reflection of light should be located in exactly the same position in each iris.

29. _____ Before referral, it is important to retest any child exhibiting an abnormality on a vision screening test.

30. _____ A child, aged 5 and enrolled in kindergarten, should be referred if he or she tests 20/30 in one eye on the Snellen E chart.

31. _____ A report of 20/50 on a Snellen E chart means that the right eye was able to read the letters on the chart at 20 feet and the left eye could read them at 50 feet.

32. _____ In administering the cover test to children over 6 months of age, the examiner would note a deviation from normal if there was a jerking movement of the eye when the cover was removed.

33. _____ The cover test is used to evaluate coloboma.

34. _____ Reevaluation or referral would be indicated for the child, aged 6, who cannot accurately identify the colors black, red, blue, yellow, and green.

The internal eyes

35. On Fig. 4-3, label the following:
    a. Arteries
    b. Veins
    c. Optic disk
    d. Physiologic cup
    e. Macula
    f. Fovea centralis

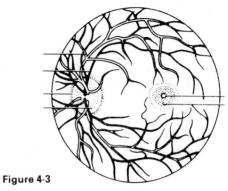

Figure 4-3

36. The elevated optic disk of papilledema is measured in _____.
37. Lesions of the retina are measured in relationship to the optic disk size,

    in terms of_____ _____.

38. The color of the optic disk is normally_____.
39. The hyperopic eye requires (*plus, minus*) adjustment of the lenses of the ophthalmoscope.
40. The myopic eye requires (*plus, minus*) adjustment of the ophthalmoscope.

41. The lens of the eye can be visualized at a setting of _____

    to _____.

42. Papilledema is a sign of _____ _____ _____.
43. The narrowing or blocking of a vein where an arteriole crosses over is termed

    _____.

44. The blurring of margins of the disk is due to _____.
45. The normal ratio of retinal arteries to veins is _____._____.
46. The macula is located (*nasally, temporally*) from the optic nerve.

HEALTH HISTORY AND ASSESSMENT

If the answer is yes, place a check (✔) at the left and provide further information in the Remarks column.

Adult Health History: Head and Neck, Part 1

Remarks

_____ Any disturbance in vision?
_____ Spots?
_____ Double vision?
_____ Halo around lights?
_____ Intolerance to lights?
_____ Visual changes?
_____ Wear glasses? Where obtained?
_____ Pain, burning, itching?
_____ Redness or discharge?
_____ Swelling of lids?
_____ Headaches?
_____ Eye problems (glaucoma, cataract, stye, infection)?
_____ Date of last eye examination?

Adult Eye Physical Assessment

Check (✔) if normal, _NE_ if not examined, _X_ if abnormal. Describe abnormal findings.

Description

_____ Eyes, brows, and lids: good alignment, symmetrical
_____ Lids: no lid lag, no inflamation or edema
_____ Sclera: white
_____ Conjunctiva: pink, noninflamed
_____ Lacrimal glands: nontender
_____ Iris: round, intact
_____ PERRLA
_____ Normal visual fields (N.II)
_____ Convergence within 5 to 8 cm
_____ Extraocular movements intact (N.III, N.IV, N.VI)

_____ Visual acuity:

Corrected: OD_____ OS_____

Uncorrected: OD_____ OS_____

_____ Corneal reflex intact (N.V)

_____ Cornea, lens: no opacities

_____ Fundi:

    _____ Optic disks: flat, yellow, margins clear

    _____ Physiologic cup flat

    _____ Arteries, veins: normal ratio

    _____ No AV nicking, hemorrhage, or exudate

Recommendations, treatment, or disposition of abnormal findings:

Geriatric Adaptations— History

Description

_____ Any visual problems?

    _____ Duration?

    _____ Sudden or gradual?

    _____ In one or both eyes?

_____ Difficulty with vision at night?

_____ Difficulty with reading small print?

_____ Require more light to read?

_____ Farsighted? Hold reading material farther away?

_____ Difficulty in distinguishing between blues, greens, and purples?

_____ Halos around lights?

    Are those glasses yours?

_____ When were your eyes last examined by a doctor?

Physical

_____ Diminished central vision; turns head slightly to use peripheral vision

_____ Pupil size diminished

_____ Cloudiness of lens (examine with +12 to +15 diopter and slowly decrease positivity until retina is seen)

_____ Opaque white ring around periphery of cornea

_____ Farsighted

Pediatric Adaptation— History

Remarks

_____ Child premature?

_____ Oxygen administered at birth?

_____ Frequent blinking?

_____ Trouble seeing?

_____ Problems with schoolwork because of difficulty seeing?

_____ Pain in the eye?

_____ Frequent squinting?

_____ Holding book closer than 12 in to read?

_____ Eyes not straight?

_____ Cross-eyes?

_____ Injury or trauma to eye?

_____ Injury or trauma to head?

_____ Migraine headaches accompanied by visual changes?

_____ Confusion or difficulty identifying colors (beyond age 5)?

_____ Family history of ptosis of eyelid?

Pediatric Adaptation— Physical

Description

_____ Normal shape in accordance with ethnic origin

_____ No abnormal slant

_____ No dark circles under eyes

_____ No sunken eyeballs or eye sockets

_____ Eyes exhibit expression, are not blank

_____ No edema of lids (in infants, should rapidly disappear after birth)

_____ Eyelashes present

_____ No abnormal coloration of eyelashes

_____ Ectropion/entropion not present

_____ No ptosis of lids

_____ No retraction of upper lid

_____ No excessive or decreased tearing

_____ Tearing present past 3 months

_____ No photophobia

_____ No exophthalmos/enophthalmos

_____ No hypertelorism/hypotelorism

_____ No nystagmus beyond 4 months

_____ No setting-sun sign

_____ Blinks approximately every 10 seconds

_____ Full ROM of ocular muscles

_____ Color of iris _____ (color set between 6 and 12 months)

_____ No dulling of color of iris

_____ No irregularity in shape of iris

_____ No Brushfield's spots on iris

_____ No anisocoria

_____ No exceptionally large/small pupil

_____ Pupils equal and react to light

_____ No cataract/opacity of lens

_____ No dislocation of lens

Vision

Infant

_____ Blinks in response to presentation of light

_____ Direct or consensual pupillary response in response to light

_____ Blinks in response to object moved rapidly toward eyes

1 to 3 months

_____ Follows bright objects with eyes for 180° range

_____ Tear glands respond to emotion

_____ Responds to bright colors and lights

3 to 4 months

_____ Able to focus on hands

_____ Can fixate on objects beyond 3 feet

4 to 7 months

_____ Displays eye-hand coordination

_____ Prefers red and yellow DDST blocks

_____ Hand-eye coordination evident (child can pick up dropped object)

7 to 11 months

_____ Can fixate on small objects and tries to pick them up

12 to 18 months

_____ Discriminates among simple geometric forms

_____ Stares at patterns

_____ Results of Denver Eye Screening Test (infants and preschoolers): Right eye _____

Left eye _____

Age 3 and beyond

_____ Results of Snellen E screening test: Right eye_____

Left eye_____

_____ No abnormality in Hirshberg's test

_____ No abnormality in cover test

_____ Beyond age 4, identifies colors with color blocks

_____ Map visual fields

_____ (3 to 5 years) Peripheral vision at 90° angle

_____ (Older child) Reads holding book no closer than 1 foot from eyes

Ethnic Adaptation— Physical

Oriental client

Description

_____ Entropion (within normal limits)

_____ Presence of epicanthal folds in Oriental infants

_____ Presence of Mongolian fold (horizontal fold in upper eyelid)

Black client

_____ Sclera may appear slightly brownish

_____ Fundus of eye may be darker than orange-red

Student_____

INSTRUCTOR'S GUIDE FOR EVALUATION OF STUDENT PERFORMANCE

Assessment of the eyes (except ophthalmoscopy)

Behaviors evaluated	Yes	No	Remarks
1. Assembles equipment needed			
2. Takes appropriate history pertinent to eyes and vision			
3. Asks branching questions as appropriate			
4. Explains procedure for examination to client			
5. Checks vision correctly using Snellen eye chart			
6. Places client in sitting position on examining table			
7. Checks eyes, lids, and brows for alignment, symmetry			
8. Depresses lower lid to observe conjunctiva and sclera			
9. Checks EOM through six cardinal fields of gaze			
10. Checks for lid lag			
11. Checks visual fields			
12. Checks convergence			
13. With oblique lighting, checks cornea and lens			
14. Checks corneal reflex			
15. Using a penlight in dim light, checks direct and consensual pupillary constriction			
16. Checks accommodation			
17. Records findings, using appropriate terminology			

Instructor: _____ Date _____

Student_____

INSTRUCTOR'S GUIDE FOR EVALUATION OF STUDENT PERFORMANCE

Assessment of the internal eye

Behaviors evaluated	Yes	No	Remarks
1. Assembles equipment needed			
2. Explains procedure for examination to client			
3. Positions client in sitting position on examining table			
4. Darkens room			
5. Turns on ophthalmoscope to brightest light			
6. Selects large aperture of the ophthalmoscope			
7. Sets the lens at 0			
8. Positions self at eye level with client			
9. Holds ophthalmoscope correctly			
a. Holds ophthalmoscope in right hand in front of own right eye			
b. Positions self at client's right side			
10. Instructs client to stare straight ahead at an object across the room			
11. At a distance of approximately 12 in in front and 25° to the right side of client, directs light beam into the pupil and locates the red reflex			
12. Slowly moves toward client, rotating lenses with right forefinger			
13. Focuses on near objects by rotating lenses to positive numbers (+15 to +20)			
14. Focuses on retina by rotating lenses to 0 (or plus or minus numbers as needed for clear focus on structure)			
15. Examines retina in the following sequence:			
a. Optic disk			
b. Retinal vessels			
c. Retinal background			
d. Macular area			

Behaviors evaluated	Yes	No	Remarks
16. Holds ophthalmoscope in left hand in front of own left eye			
17. Positions self at client's left side			
18. Repeats examination for the left eye			
19. Correctly describes these findings:			
a. Lens			
b. Disk			
c. Retinal background			
d. Vessels			
e. Macular area			
20. Records findings, using appropriate medical terminology			

Instructor: _____ Date _____

MODULE 5

ASSESSMENT OF THE HEAD AND NECK, PART 2 (EAR)

This instructional module is designed as a guide to assist you in learning a thorough and systematic approach to assessment of the ear, including auditory acuity and the use of the otoscope. Adaptation for assessing the infant, child, and geriatric client are included. Some ethnic variations are also covered. You are to complete this module and pass the Posttest before the scheduled laboratory period for assessment of the head and neck, part 2.

If you have difficulty in completing this module, contact your instructor.

PREREQUISITE OBJECTIVES

You should be able to:

1. Label the anatomical structures on a diagram of the ear.
2. Label the major landmarks on a diagram of the tympanic membrane.
3. Describe the functions of the middle and inner ear.
4. Describe the physiology of hearing.

TERMINAL OBJECTIVES

Upon completion of this module you are expected to be able to:

1. Define the vocabulary words accompanying this module.
2. Take a health history pertinent to the ears and hearing, using appropriate branching questions.
3. Describe guidelines for evaluating the alignment and position of the ears.
4. Demonstrate the correct use of an otoscope.

115

5. Describe the appearance of the normal tympanic membrane.

6. Demonstrate Rinne's test for hearing loss.

7. Demonstrate Weber's test for hearing loss.

8. Describe a method for testing gross auditory acuity in the infant, preschool child, and adult.

9. Identify common behavioral patterns in the child which could indicate a hearing deficit.

10. Describe the sweep-check screening test for assessing hearing loss.

11. Describe the arousal test used to assess gross hearing of a newborn.

12. Describe the orienting-response-to-noise test for assessing hearing acuity of infants.

13. Describe the anatomical differences in the structures of the ear among the infant, child, and adult that will be of significance to the examiner.

14. Describe the hearing changes that can occur with aging.

15. Perform an assessment of the ears, using an assessment form as a guide.

16. Record the data obtained from the health assessment using correct medical terminology.

SUGGESTED ACTIVITIES

Read

Bates, Barbara: "The Ear" and "Pediatric Physical Examination: The Ear," *A Guide to Physical Examination,* Lippincott, Philadelphia, 1979.

OR

Malasanos, Lois, et al.: "The Ear" and "Assessment of the Pediatric Client: The Ear," *Health Assessment,* Mosby, St. Louis, 1977.

Caird, F.I., and T. G. Judge: "The Ear," *Assessment of the Elderly Patient,* Pitman, California, 1977.

OR

Saxon, Sue V., and Mary Jean Etten: "The Sensory Systems: Hearing Audition," *Physical Change and Aging,* The Tiresias Press, New York, 1978.

Alexander, Mary, and Marie Brown: "Ears," *Pediatric History Taking and Physical Diagnosis for Nurses,* McGraw-Hill, New York, 1979.

OR

Brown, Marie S., and Mary M. Alexander: "Physical Examination: Part 7, Examining the Ears," *Nursing '74,* 48-51 (February, 1974).

Mead Johnson Company: *The Ears,* Evansville, Ill. (newborn).

View

Examining the External and Middle Ear, Concept Media video cassette, 29 min.
Assessing Hearing—Children, Concept Media video cassette, 27 min.

Equipment
otoscope
tuning fork no. 256

PRETEST   With books closed, test your knowledge of anatomy and physiology of the ear.

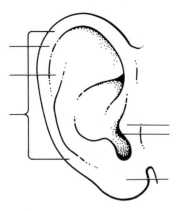

Figure 5-1

1. Using Fig. 5-1, label the following:
   a. Helix
   b. Antihelix
   c. Tragus
   d. Auditory canal
   e. Lobe
   f. Auricle or pinna

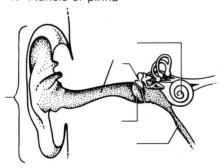

Figure 5-2

2. Using Fig. 5-2, label the following:
   a. Cochlea
   b. Eustachian tube
   c. Ossicles (malleus, incus, stapes)
   d. Tympanic membrane
   e. Auricle
   f. Auditory canal

3. The cranial nerve that contols hearing and balance is the _____
nerve.

4. Describe the function of the malleus, incus, and stapes.

5. List two functions of the ear.

VOCABULARY

audiometer	mastoid	pars flaccida	stapes
cerumen	otalgia	pars tensa	tragus
cochlea	otitis externa	pinna	umbo
eustachian tube	otitis media	presbycusis	vertigo
incus	otodynia	Rinne's test	Weber's test
malleus	otorrhea	serous otitis	

DECISION TABLE 5-1

If . . .   **Then . . .**

You are interested in color photo- ⟹ Abbott Laboratories: *Atlas of Some
graphs of pathology of the eardrum   Pathological Conditions of the Eye,
and canal   Ear, Throat.*

You like programmed instruction ⟹ Mechner, Francis: "Patient Assess-
                                                                 ment: Examination of the Ear,"
                                                                 American Journal of Nursing, **75**(3):,
                                                                 (March, 1975).

You need more information on assess- ⟹ Brown, Marie S., and Mary M.
ing hearing acuity   Alexander: "Physical Examination,
                                                                 Part 8, Hearing Acuity," *Nursing '73,*
                                                                 61–65 (April, 1973) (excellent on hear-
                                                                 ing tests for infants and children; in-
                                                                 cludes audiometry).

                                                  ⟹ Payne, Peter D., and Regina L.
                                                                 Payne: "Behavior Manifestations in
                                                                 Children with Hearing Loss," *Ameri-
                                                                 can Journal of Nursing,* 1718–1719
                                                                 (August, 1970).

You need help with history taking ⟹ Wasson, John, et al.: *Common
and suggestions for physical examina-   Symptom Guide,* McGraw-Hill, 1975.
tion for specific ear problems

You desire additional or alternate ⟹ *Pediatric Physical Examination—Ear,
media   Nose, Mouth, and Throat,* Blue-Hill
                                                                 Educational Systems, videotape, 53
                                                                 min.

DECISION TABLE 5-1 (continued)

If . . .		Then . . .
	⟹	*Physical Assessment Examination— Ear, Nose, Mouth, and Throat,* Blue-Hill Educational Systems, videotape, 19 min.
You wish additional pediatric references	⟹	Barness, Lewis A.: *Manual of Pediatric Physical Diagnosis,* Year Book, Chicago, 1972, pp. 66-74.
	⟹	Chinn, Peggy L., and Cynthia Leitch: *Child Health Maintenance: A Guide to Clinical Assessment,* Mosby, St. Louis, 2d ed., 1979, pp. 35-36.

POSTTEST

1. The color of the normal tympanic membrane is:
   a. Pink
   b. White
   c. Gray
   d. Amber

2. To straighten the ear canal in the older child and adult, the pinna should be pulled

   _____ and _____ .

3. To straighten the ear canal in the infant and young child, the pinna should be

   pulled _____ and _____ .

Match

4. _____ Client in light sleep before the test

5. _____ A test for lateralization, using a tuning fork

6. _____ A test comparing air and bone conduction

7. _____ A hearing test in which the audiometer is used

8. _____ A frequently employed method for gross testing of hearing in an older child or adult

a. Rinne's test
b. Weber's test
c. Sweep-check test
d. Ticking watch
e. Arousal test
f. Orienting-response-to-noise test

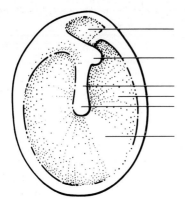

Figure 5-3

9. Using Fig. 5-3, label the following:
   a. Pars flaccida
   b. Pars tensa
   c. Cone of light
   d. Umbo
   e. Handle of malleus
   f. Short process of malleus

10. The ossicle attached to the tympanic membrane is the
    a. Malleus
    b. Incus
    c. Stapes

11. List *five* observations of the external canal that should be noted in examining the ear.

    a. _____

    b. _____

    c. _____

    d. _____

    e. _____

12. Describe *one* way to determine if ears are low set in relation to the eyes.

13. List *four* behaviors of a 2-year-old that could indicate a hearing loss.

a. _____

b. _____

c. _____

d. _____

Write *true* or *false.* If *false,* correct the statement to make it true.

14. _____ Malformations in the shape of the infant's ear may indicate malformations of other organ systems or chromosomal alterations.

15. _____ The ears have attained adult size by the age of 6.

16. _____ The presence of Darwin's tubercle on the helix of the ear represents pathology.

17. _____ Low-set ears often indicate pathology.

18. _____ Half the persons over 65 have some hearing loss.

19. _____ In age-related hearing loss, the low-frequency sounds are usually affected first.

20. _____ One of the most common causes of problems with the ear in the child is the presence of a foreign body in the ear.

21. _____ The examiner is often alerted to hearing problems in a child when a history of poor school performance is elicited.

22. _____ A diffuse light reflex on the tympanic membrane of an infant should alert the examiner to a defect.

23. _____ Referral would be indicated when dry, gray, brittle earwax is found in the ear of an Oriental client.

In examination of the ear with an otoscope, you discover the following findings. Write *yes* for the findings which are significant and warrant referral and *no* for the insignificant or normal findings.

24. _____ White, chalky patches on the tympanic membrane

25. _____ Air bubbles behind the tympanic membrane

26. _____ Dark brown cerumen

27. _____ Pearly gray tympanic membrane

28. _____ No visible bony landmarks

29. _____ No cone of light

30. _____ Hairline air-fluid level

31. _____ Visible handle and short process of the malleus

32. _____ Retracted tympanic membrane

33. _____ Hyperemic vessels across tympanic membrane

HEALTH HISTORY AND ASSESSMENT

If the answer is yes, place a check (✔) at the left and provide further information in the Remarks column.

Adult Health History: Head and Neck, Part 2

Remarks

_____ Hard of hearing?
_____ When were ears last examined?
_____ Constant ringing or buzzing in ears?
_____ Chronic running ear?
_____ Chronic ear infections?
_____ Earaches with colds or plane flights?
_____ Ears stopped-up?
_____ Chronic itching?
_____ Loss of equilibrium?
_____ Vertigo or dizziness?
_____ Changes in hearing?
_____ Noisy environment?

Adult Ear Physical Assessment

Check (✔) if normal, *NE* if not examined, *X* if abnormal. Describe abnormal findings.

Description

_____ Symmetrical
_____ Correct alignment with eyes
_____ Auricle: No masses or tenderness
_____ Canal: No lesions or discharge
_____ Cerumen present and of quality appropriate to ethnic origin
_____ Tympanic membrane: Clear, intact, good light reflex, all landmarks present
_____ Auditory acuity (N.VIII) normal to ticking watch or whisper
_____ Weber: Lateralizes equally
_____ Rinne: AC is greater than BC

Geriatric Adaptations— History

_____ Any difficulty with hearing?

_____ How long ago?

_____ Was it sudden?

_____ Wear a hearing aid?

_____ Is the hearing aid yours?

_____ Date of last hearing test?

_____ Difficulty with hearing high-frequency sounds?

_____ Ears stopped-up?

_____ Difficulty with equilibrium or balance?

Physical

Description

_____ Diminished hearing, especially high-frequency sounds

_____ Thickened cerumen

_____ Thickened tympanic membranes

_____ Diminished sense of equilibrium, especially if moving rapidly

Pediatric Adaptations— History

Remarks

_____ History of deafness in family?

_____ Frequent ear infections/otitis media?

_____ History of rubella of mother in first trimester of pregnancy?

_____ Prematurity or low birth weight?

_____ Prolonged hospitalization at birth?

_____ Jaundice during first week of life?

_____ History of cleft lip or cleft palate?

_____ History of speech difficulty?

_____ History of foreign bodies in ear?

_____ Problems with progress in school?

_____ Seems unable to hear?

_____ Does not turn to source of noise?

_____ Does not respond to commands or name?

_____ Turns radio or television volume too high?

_____ Speaks in a loud or monotonous tone?

_____ Rubs or pulls at ears?

Physical   Description

Infant

_____ Arouses from sleep with sudden noise (0 to 3 months of age)

_____ Responds to sudden, sharp, sound by blinking eyes

_____ Turns head or eyes to localize sounds of tinkling bell

_____ Eyes wide, turns head slightly (4 to 5 months)

_____ Turns head toward sound (6 to 7 months)

_____ Turns head toward sound and can determine whether the sound is above or below

_____ Responds to name (6 to 10 months)

_____ Imitates simple words (10 to 15 months)

_____ Light reflex on tympanic membrane diffuse (infant)

Child

_____ Responds to watch test or whispered sounds

_____ No malformation of ears

_____ Tip of pinna on horizontal line running from outer canthus of eye to occipital protuberance

_____ Light cone present (child)

_____ No unusual odors

_____ No foreign bodies

_____ No enlargement of postauricular nodes

_____ No abnormality of vestibular
function

_____ Results of audiometric screening test, if administered:
R ear _____ L ear _____

**Ethnic
Adaptations—
Physical**

American Indian or Oriental client   Description

_____ Earwax dry

_____ Earwax gray and brittle

Black and Caucasian clients

_____ Earwax wet

_____ Earwax brown and sticky

Student_____

INSTRUCTOR'S GUIDE FOR EVALUATION OF STUDENT PERFORMANCE

Assessment of the Ears

Behaviors evaluated	Yes	No	Remarks
1. Assembles equipment needed			
2. Takes appropriate history pertinent to the ears and hearing			
3. Asks branching questions as appropriate			
4. Explains procedure for examination to the client			
5. Places client in sitting position on the examining table			
6. Inspects external ear and mastoid			
7. Checks alignment of eyes with ears			
8. Checks auditory acuity with ticking watch or whisper			
9. Performs Weber's test accurately			
10. Performs Rinne's test accurately			
11. Straightens ear canal			
12. Uses otoscope correctly			
13. Correctly describes these findings:			
a. Color of tympanic membrane			
b. Landmarks			
c. Light reflex			
d. Lesions, cerumen, foreign objects or exudate			
e. Redness or edema of canal			
14. Records findings, using appropriate terminology			

Instructor _____ Date _____

MODULE 6

ASSESSMENT OF THE HEAD AND NECK, PART 3 (HEAD, NECK, NOSE, SINUSES, AND ORAL CAVITY)

This instructional module is designed as a guide to assist you in learning a thorough and systematic approach for assessment of the head, neck, nose, sinuses, and oral cavity. Assessment of the head and neck is divided into three modules. Parts 1 and 2 precede this module and includes assessment of the eye and ear. As in previous modules, emphasis is on taking an appropriate health history and performing a thorough examination. Adaptations for assessing the infant, child, and geriatric client and ethnic variations are included. You are to complete this module and pass the Posttest before the scheduled laboratory period.

If you have difficulty in completing the module, contact your instructor.

PREREQUISITE OBJECTIVES
You should be able to:

1. Label the major structures on a diagram of the head.
2. Label the major bones, fontanels, and sutures on a diagram of the head of an infant.
3. Label the major anatomical structures on a diagram of the oral cavity.
4. Label the teeth on a diagram of the deciduous and permanent teeth.
5. State the age at which eruption of the teeth occurs.
6. Label the major anatomical structures on a diagram of the neck.
7. List the names and functions of the cranial nerves.

129

TERMINAL OBJECTIVES

Upon completion of this module you are expected to be able to:

1. Define the vocabulary words accompanying this module.
2. Given an assessment form as a guide, take a health history pertinent to the head and neck, using appropriate branching questions.
3. Demonstrate the correct use of a nasal speculum.
4. Demonstrate palpation of the frontal and maxillary sinuses.
5. Demonstrate palpation of the trachea for deviation.
6. Demonstrate one procedure for assessing the thyroid gland.
7. Name and locate the lymph nodes that drain the head and neck.
8. Demonstrate the correct procedure for testing cranial nerves I, V, VII, IX, X, XI, and XII.
9. Demonstrate the correct procedure for assessment of the head, face, neck, nose, sinuses, mouth, and pharynx, using an assessment form as a guide.
10. Demonstrate variation of techniques used in examination of the child.
11. Describe the anatomical differences of the head and neck among the newborn, child, and adult that are of significance to the examiner.
12. Describe the changes in the ability to taste and smell that can occur with aging.
13. Describe variations in the physical characteristics of the head and neck that may occur among ethnic groups.
14. Record the data obtained from the health assessment using correct medical terminology

SUGGESTED ACTIVITIES

Read

Alexander, Mary M., and Marie Scott Brown: "Nose, Mouth, and Throat" and "Lymphatics," *Pediatric History Taking and Physical Diagnosis for Nurses,* McGraw-Hill, New York, 1979.

OR

Chinn, Peggy L., and Cynthia Leitch: *Child Health Maintenance: A Guide to Clinical Assessment,* Mosby, St. Louis, 2d ed., 1979.

Bates, Barbara: "Head and Neck," *A Guide to Physical Examination,* Lippincott, Philadelphia, 1979.

OR

Malasanos, Lois, et al: "Nose, Throat, Head, Face and Neck," *Health Assessment,* Mosby, St. Louis, 1977.

Caird, F. I., and T. G. Judge: "Head and Neck," *Assessment of the Elderly Patient,* Pitman, California, 1976.

OR

Saxon, Sue V., and Mary Jean Etten: "The Sensory Systems," *Physical Change and Aging,* The Tiresias Press, New York, 1978.

View

Bates, Barbara: *Examination of the Head and Neck,* Lippincott, videotape, 14.5 min.

Biologic Changes of Aging: Physical Assessment and Special Senses, Trainex program 453, frames 45-83.

Physical Examination of the School-Age Child—Oral Cavity, Trainex program 502.

Equipment

penlight
tongue depressor
nasal speculum
centimeter tape measure
glove
stethoscope

If neurological examination is included:

cotton
safety pin

PRETEST

1. On Fig. 6-1, label the following:

   a. Frontal bone
   b. Nasal bone
   c. Maxilla
   d. Mandible
   e. Zygomatic bone
   f. Occipital bone

   g. Temporal bone
   h. Mastoid process
   i. Parietal bone
   j. Parotid gland and duct
   k. Submaxillary gland and duct

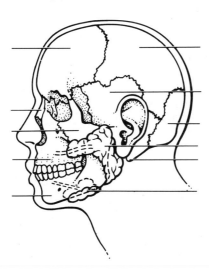

Figure 6-1

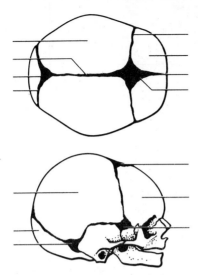

Figure 6-2

2. On Fig. 6-2, label the following:
   a. Sagittal suture
   b. Coronal suture
   c. Frontal suture
   d. Lambdoid suture
   e. Anterior fontanel
   f. Sphenoid fontanel

   g. Mastoid fontanel
   h. Posterior fontanel
   i. Parietal bone
   j. Frontal bone
   k. Occipital bone

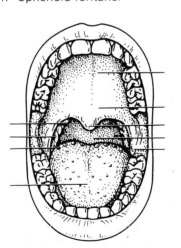

Figure 6-3

3. On Fig. 6-3, label the following:
   a. Soft palate
   b. Hard palate
   c. Uvula
   d. Tonsil
   e. Anterior pillar

   f. Posterior pillar
   g. Posterior pharyngeal wall
   h. Vallate papilla
   i. Dorsum of tongue

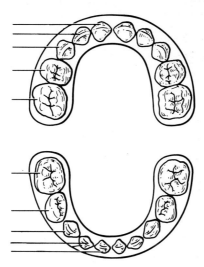

Figure 6-4

4. On Fig. 6-4, label the following deciduous teeth and age at eruption:
   a. Central incisor
   b. Lateral incisor
   c. Cuspid
   d. First molar
   e. Second molar

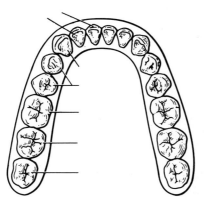

Figure 6-5

5. On Fig. 6-5, label the following permanent teeth:
   a. Central incisor   e. First molar
   b. Lateral incisor   f. Second molar
   c. Cuspid   g. Third molar
   d. Bicuspids

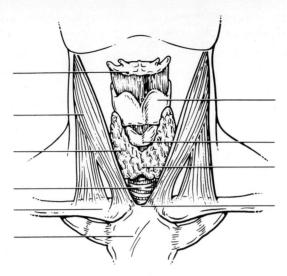

Figure 6-6

6. On Fig. 6-6, label the following:

   a. Clavicle
   b. Trachea
   c. Manubrium of sternum
   d. Sternal notch
   e. Sternocleidomastoid muscle

   f. Hyoid bone
   g. Thyroid cartilage
   h. Cricoid cartilage
   i. Lobe of thyroid
   j. Isthmus of thyroid

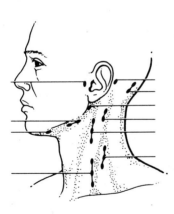

Figure 6-7

7. On Fig. 6-7, label the lymph nodes:

   a. Preauricular
   b. Postauricular
   c. Occipital
   d. Tonsillar
   e. Submandibular (Submaxillary)

   f. Submental
   g. Anterior cervical
   h. Posterior cervical
   i. Supraclavicular

8. Match the following cranial nerves with the appropriate name and function. (Include all appropriate functions.)

Name	Function	Name	Function
I ____	____	a. Facial	1. Jaw movement
V ____	____	b. Glosso-pharyngeal	2. Movement of tongue
VII ____	____	c. Hypoglossal	3. Movement of facial muscles
IX ____	____	d. Olfactory	4. Movement of palate, pharynx, larynx
X ____	____	e. Spinal accessory	5. Smell
XI ____	____	f. Trigeminal	6. Sensation in ophthalmic, maxillary, mandibular areas of face
XII ____	____	g. Vagus	7. Taste on anterior two-thirds of tongue

8. Sensation on posterior tongue and pharynx, gag reflex
9. Sensation in pharynx, larynx
10. Sternocleidomastoid muscle movement
11. Corneal reflex

VOCABULARY

Descriptive terminology

adenoids, bruit, buccal, caries, cryptic, dysphagia, edentulous, epistaxis, fontanel, frenulum, gingivitis, glossitis, grimace, hypertelorism, hypotelorism, lymphadenopathy, macrocephalic, macroglossia, microcephalic, micrognathia, normocephalic, papillae, parotid gland, pharyngitis, polyp, rhinitis, Stensen's duct, stomatitis, turbinate, uvula, Wharton's duct

Diagnostic terminology

Brudzinski's sign, canker, caput succedaneum, cephalhematoma, chancre, cheilitis, craniotabes, Epstein's pearls, geographic tongue, goiter, herpes simplex, Hutchinson's teeth, hydrocephalic, leukoplakia, moniliasis, opisthotonos, periodontitis, thrush

---

DECISION TABLE 6-1

If . . .		Then . . .
You need well-illustrated newborn and infant references	⟹	Mead Johnson Company, *The Mouth and the Head*, Evansville, Ill.
You prefer programmed instruction	⟹	Mechner, Francis: "Patient Assessment: Examination of the Head and Neck," *American Journal of Nursing*, 75(5), (May, 1975).
You need help with general descriptors and branching questions for history taking and suggestions for physical examination	⟹	Wasson, John, et al.: "Mouth Problems and Nose-Sinus Trouble," *The Common Symptom Guide*, McGraw-Hill, New York, 1975.
You are interested in a thorough dental history	⟹	Slattery, Jill: "Dental Health in Children," *American Journal of Nursing*, 1159-1161 (July, 1976) (A dental history form is included.)
	⟹	Dyer, Elaine D., et al.: "Dental Health in Adults," *American Journal of Nursing*, 1156-1158 (July, 1976).
You need more information on oral cancer screening	⟹	Keough, Gertrude, and Harold N. Niebel: "Oral Cancer Detection — A Nursing Responsibility," *American Journal of Nursing*, 684-686 (April, 1973). (Describes signs and symptoms of oral cancer and methods of detection; several color illustrations.)
You desire additional or alternative media	⟹	*Pediatric Examination — Ear, Nose, Throat, and Mouth*, Blue-Hill Educational System videotape, 53 min.
	⟹	*Physical Assessment Examination — Ear, Nose, Throat, and Mouth*, Blue-Hill Educational System videotape, 19 min.

POSTTEST   Match the definitions with the correct terms.

1. _____ Inflammation of the gums
2. _____ Without teeth
3. _____ Small lower jaw
4. _____ Large tongue
5. _____ Inflammation of tongue
6. _____ Enlarged thyroid
7. _____ Deep, irregular crevices

a. Cryptic
b. Micrognathia
c. Macroglossia
d. Gingivitis
e. Glossitis
f. Goiter
g. Periodontitis
h. Edentulous
i. Geographic tongue

8. List *three* pertinent observations of the face.

    a. _____

    b. _____

    c. _____

9. The teeth and gums should be inspected for

    a. _____

    b. _____

    c. _____

    d. _____

10. A thin white coating on the tongue is considered to be
    a. An indication of dietary deficiency
    b. A yeast infection
    c. Leukoplakia
    d. Normal for most people

11. Tonsils should be inspected for

    a. _____

    b. _____

    c. _____

    d. _____

12. Lymph nodes should be assessed for

    a. _____

    b. _____

    c. _____

    d. _____

13. An enlarged thyroid gland should be auscultated for _____.

14. Swallowing will cause the thyroid gland to
    a. Rise
    b. Stay the same while the trachea rises
    c. Fall

15. Name the *two* fontanels that are easily palpated in the infant.

    a. _____

    b. _____

16. The normal head size of an infant at birth is approximately _____ cm.

17. In the newborn, is the head *larger* or *smaller* than the chest? _____

18. All deciduous teeth have usually erupted at age _____.

Write *true* or *false*. Correct the false statements to make them true.

19. _____ The nasal mucosa is usually a little deeper red than the oral mucosa.

20. _____ The three nasal turbinates are visible with a wide nasal speculum.

21. _____ The ethmoid, maxillary, and frontal sinuses are present at birth.

22. _____ Sinus tenderness is determined by pressing upward against the sinus areas.

23. _____ The frontal and maxillary sinuses are the only sinuses readily accessible for examination.

24. _____ The thyroid gland may be palpated from the front or the back of the client.

25. _____ Normal-sized lateral lobes of the thyroid are usually palpable.

26. _____ The isthmus of the thyroid is usually palpable.

27. _____ The measurement of the circumference of the head should be a part of the routine examination of an infant or child.

28. _____ The sensation of taste is markedly decreased in many elderly clients.

29. _____ The ability to smell decreases markedly with aging.

30. _____ Atrophy of the papillae at the sides of the tongue is common in the elderly.

31. _____ Inspection of the mouth should be performed with the dentures in place.

32. _____ The thyroid gland is usually not palpable in the elderly.

Match each diagnostic technique with the cranial nerve being tested:

33. _____ Shrugs shoulders
34. _____ Says "ah"
35. _____ Smiles, grimaces
36. _____ Protrudes tongue
37. _____ Clenches teeth

a. Trigeminal
b. Facial
c. Glossopharyngeal
d. Vagus
e. Spinal accessory
f. Hypoglossal

In performing a health assessment, you discover the following findings. Write *yes* for the findings which are significant and warrant referral and *no* for the insignificant or normal findings.

38. _____ A young adult with patches of red, denuded areas on the dorsum of the tongue.

39. _____ An adolescent with visible, cryptic tonsils.

40. _____ A newborn infant with white, curdlike patches on the buccal mucosa.

41. _____ A child with mottled, discolored teeth.

42. _____ A young adult with an enlarged thyroid gland.

43. _____ An adult with lymphoid patches of tissue on the posterior pharyngeal wall.

Write *true* or *false.* Correct the false statements to make them true.

44. _____ In a child, a flattened nose and deviated septum may be indicative of cleft palate.

45. _____ Unilateral purulent nasal secretions in a child may prompt the examiner to check for the presence of a foreign body in the nose.

46. _____ It is not unusual for the child to breath through the mouth.

47. _____ The head shape of a child is noted by observing the child from the front.

48. _____ Head circumference is measured by running the tape over the occipital protuberance to the midforehead.

49. _____ The examiner usually has no difficulty examining the mouth of a child.

50. _____ In the young infant (below 3 months), epithelial pearls may normally be found in or near the midline of the gums.

51. _____ If a child cannot elevate the tip of the tongue to make sounds like *t, d,* and *n,* then the child must be referred for evaluation of a shortened frenulum.

52. _____ Presence of a high arched palate in a child may indicate chronic mouth breathing.

53. _____ Tonsils in the child are normally enlarged as compared with the tonsils of an adult.

54. _____ The correct way to record the size of the anterior fontanel is: "anterior fontanel 3 cm."

55. _____ Bulging fontanels are a sign of dehydration in the infant.

56. _____ Presence of a foreign body in the trachea of a child may be indicated by a palpatory thud felt or heard over the trachea.

57. _____ Palpation of an additional horizontal suture in the occiput of an American Indian child would be a normal finding.

58. _____ Craniotabes are a normal finding in children up to age 6.

HEALTH HISTORY AND ASSESSMENT

Adult Health History: Head and Neck, Part 3

If the answer is yes, place a check (✔) at the left and provide further information in the Remarks column.

Head and neck   Remarks

_____ Severe headaches or head pains?

_____ Dizziness or fainting?

_____ Head injury?

_____ Pain or stiffness in neck?

_____ Swelling or enlarged glands?

_____ Goiter or thyroid trouble?

_____ Need to take thyroid medicine?

Nose and sinuses

_____ Chronic stuffy or runny nose?

_____ Loss of smell?

_____ Chronic drip from nose to throat?

_____ Frequently use nose drops?

_____ Nosebleeds?

Mouth and throat

_____ Frequent colds or sore throat?

_____ Need to clear throat frequently?

_____ Hoarseness at times?

_____ Any known dental problems?

_____ Wear dentures, partial plates, or braces?

_____ Proper fit?

_____ Teeth extractions?

_____ More than a year since teeth checked?

_____ Sore mouth or tongue?

_____ History of mouth ulcers or fever blisters?

_____ Bad breath?

**Physical
Assessment**

Check (✔) if normal, *NE* if not examined, *X* if abnormal. Describe abnormal findings.

Head and face   Description

_____ Normocephalic, symmetrical

_____ No lumps or tenderness

_____ Normal hair distribution

_____ No lesions or dandruff

_____ Facial nerve (N. VII): Symmetri-
cal, movement intact

_____ Trigeminal nerve (N.V): Motor
and sensory, all three divisions
intact

_____ TM joint freely movable, no
pain

Nose and sinuses

_____ Mucosa and turbinates: Pink,
no discharge, polyps, or edema

_____ Septum: No deviation

_____ Patent bilaterally

_____ Sinuses: Nontender

_____ Frontal

_____ Maxillary

Mouth and pharynx

_____ Lips: No lesions or edema

_____ Teeth and gums: In good re-
pair, no obvious caries

_____ No bleeding or edema of
gums

_____ Teeth straight, even

_____ No staining or discoloration

_____ Mucous membrane: Pink, no
lesions

_____ Salivary ducts: No edema or
redness

_____ Tonsils: No crypts, enlarge-
ment, redness, or exudate

_____ Tongue: Pink, no lesions,
fasciculations or assymetry
(N.XII), frenulum present

_____ Gag reflex present (N.IX, N.X)

_____ Soft palate and uvula rise equally (N.IX, N.X)

_____ Palate intact

_____ Breath: No offensive or fruity odor

Neck

_____ Full ROM

_____ Spinal accessory (N.XI) intact, strong

_____ Trachea in midline

_____ Thyroid: Nonpalpable, no masses

_____ Salivary glands: Nontender, not enlarged

_____ Carotid pulses 4 + , equal

_____ Lymph nodes: no enlargement or tenderness

    _____ Preauricular

    _____ Postauricular

    _____ Occipital

    _____ Tonsillar

    _____ Submandibular

    _____ Submental

    _____ Anterior cervical

    _____ Posterior cervical

    _____ Supraclavicular

    _____ Infraclavicular

Geriatric Adaptations— History

_____ Has food lost its flavor?

_____ Prefer highly spiced foods?

_____ Use additional salt on food?

_____ Loss of appetite?

_____ Difficulty in swallowing?

_____ Difficulty in chewing?

_____ Dentures fit?

Physical

_____ Diminished sense of taste

_____ Diminished sense of smell

_____ No difficulty in swallowing

_____ No caries or loose, broken teeth

_____ Properly fitting dentures

_____ No lesions under dentures

_____ No leukoplakia

Recommendations, treatment, or disposition of abnormal findings:

Pediatric Adaptations— History

Remarks

_____ Head-rocking or -banging?

_____ Change in control of head?

_____ Loss of hair?

_____ Pulls out own hair?

_____ Rubs head frequently?

_____ Forceps used for delivery?

_____ Long labor with severe molding of head?

_____ Family members with genetic defects?

_____ Traumatic injury to head?

_____ Trauma to nose?

_____ Foreign body in nose?

_____ Live in high, dry altitude?

_____ Picking nose?

_____ Allergies?

_____ Exposure to chemical fumes?

_____ Snoring when sleeping?

_____ Difficulty breathing?

_____ Eats or chews paint on toys, high chairs, cribs?

_____ Frequent URI?

_____ Frequent throat infection?

_____ Removal of tonsils?

_____ Stiffness of neck?

_____ Difficulty swallowing?

_____ Vomiting? If yes, describe severity, pattern, character of vomitus

_____ Exposure to excess fluorides or tetracyclines?

_____ Injury to or traumatic loss of teeth?

_____ Frequent toothache?

_____ Problems with teething? Date of last visit to dentist?

_____

Age at onset of eruption

of teeth? _____

List months and pattern of tooth eruption (one or two teeth at a time):

Deciduous teeth: _____

Permanent teeth: _____
Presently being seen by

orthodontist?_____
Orthodontic appliances being used?

_____ Oral hygiene

How often are teeth brushed?

Who does the brushing?

Dentrifice used?

Type of toothbrush?

Pediatric Adaptations— Physical	**Head**	Description

_____ Circumference approximately 2 cm larger than chest (infant)

_____ Circumference 5 to 7 cm smaller than chest (childhood)

Circumference _____ cm

_____ Fontanels:
Anterior: Open____ closed____
    Size: _____by _____ cm
Posterior: Open____ closed____
    Size: _____by _____ cm

_____ No bulging of fontanels

_____ No marked pulsations in fontanels

_____ No dilatation of scalp veins

_____ No bruits heard over skull

_____ No sutures palpable past 6 months

_____ Describe head position when resting

_____ No head lag (past 3 months)

_____ Raises head when prone (infant)

_____ Holds head erect when sitting

_____ Pinna of ears on horizontal plane with outer canthus of eye and occipital protuberance

_____ Size of lower jaw proportional to rest of head

_____ No bulging or "bossing" of frontal area of skull

_____ Transillumination

_____ Less than 1 cm on frontal bone

_____ Minimal or absent at base of occiput

_____ No craniotabes

_____ No tenderness or pain over scalp

_____ No tenderness or pain over occiput

_____ No tenderness or pain over frontal of maxillary sinuses

Face

_____ Symmetry of facial expression

_____ Facial responses to external stimuli appropriate to age

_____ Detects touch in all facial areas

_____ Blinks in response to corneal touch

_____ Jaw movements coordinated

_____ Can mimic faces made by examiner

_____ Can discriminate among tastes presented by examiner

_____ No twitching of facial muscles

_____ No abnormal or unusual facial appearance

_____ No swelling

Mouth and throat

_____ Color of lips _____

_____ No circumoral pallor

_____ No cleft lip

_____ No lesions or fissures

_____ No unusual odors

_____ Buccal mucosa intact

_____ Well-developed sucking pods (infants)

_____ No dilatation of veins in buccal mucosa

_____ Tonsils do not occlude airway

_____ Hard palate intact

_____ Soft palate intact

_____ Palate not high, narrow, arched

_____ No abnormality of pattern of papillae or coating of tongue

_____ Color of tongue _____

_____ Tongue not enlarged or protruding

_____ No impairment in movement of tongue

_____ No shortening of frenulum (child can elevate tip of tongue to produce _t, d, n, l_ sounds)

_____ No profuse or decreased salivation

_____ No discoloration of gums

_____ Number of teeth present_____

_____ Teeth present appropriate for age

_____ No flattened edges of teeth

_____ No malocclusion

_____ No defect in tooth enamel

_____ No visible caries

_____ No staining or mottling of teeth

Larynx and pharynx

_____ Swallow reflex present

_____ No abnormality in cry

_____ No nasal speech

_____ No lisping or stuttering

_____ Pharynx clearly visible

Nose

_____ Breathes through nose; no mouth breathing

_____ Nares patent

_____ Nose shape appropriate for ethnic origin

_____ No flaring of nostrils

_____ No flattening of bridge of nose

_____ No septal deviation

_____ No foreign bodies in nose

Neck

_____ Tonic neck reflex not present after 5 months

_____ Smooth movements on head rotation

_____ No head-rolling, nodding

_____ No distention of neck veins

Ethnic Adaptations— Physical

American Indian infant   Description

_____ Presence of a horizontal suture in the occipital bone

Black client

_____ Presence of bluish pigmentation in gums

_____ Presence of freckling pigmentation in buccal cavity, gums, on borders of tongue

Student_____

INSTRUCTOR'S GUIDE FOR EVALUATION OF STUDENT PERFOR- ANCE

Assessment of the head and neck, part 3

Behaviors evaluated	Yes	No	Remarks
1. Assembles equipment needed			
2. Takes history appropriate to the head and neck*			
3. Asks appropriate branching questions*			
4. Explains examination procedure to the client			
5. Places client in sitting position on examining table (or lap of parent)			
6. Notes position of head			
7. Measures circumference of head (if a child)			
8. Inspects scalp and hair			
9. Palpates head			
10. Observes facial symmetry, expression; has client smile, grimace			
11. Tests trigeminal nerve (all three divisions), motor, sensory			
12. Palpates temporomandibular joint			
13. Inspects and palpates thyroid gland			
14. Palpates trachea			
15. Palpates carotid pulses			
16. Palpates lymph nodes			
preauricular			
postauricular			
occipital			
tonsillar			
submandibular			
submental			
anterior cervical			
posterior cervical			
supraclavicular			
infraclavicular			
17. Checks ROM of neck			
18. Checks spinal accessory nerve (has client shrug shoulders)			

*May be evaluated on previously submitted history

Behaviors evaluated	Yes	No	Remarks
19. Checks patency of nares			
20. Inspects nares with nasal speculum			
21. Palpates and percusses sinuses			
frontal			
maxillary			
22. Inspects lips			
23. Inspects teeth and gums			
24. Inspects oral mucosa			
25. Inspects salivary ducts			
26. Inspects roof of mouth			
27. Examines tongue and frenulum			
28. Checks symmetry of palate and uvula (client says "ah")			
29. Using tongue depressor, examines tonsils and pharynx			
30. Checks gag reflex			
31. Records findings, using appropriate terminology			

Instructor _____ Date _____

MODULE 7

ASSESSMENT OF THE THORAX AND LUNGS

This instructional module is designed as a guide to assist you in a thorough and systematic assessment of the thorax and lungs. Emphasis will be placed on the techniques of inspection, palpation, percussion, and auscultation of the thorax and lungs. Adaptations for assessing the infant, child, and geriatric client are included.

This module is similar in format to previous modules. You are to complete learning activities and pass the Posttest before the scheduled laboratory period for assessment of the thorax and lungs.

If you have difficulty in completing this module, contact your instructor.

PREREQUISITE OBJECTIVES

You should be able to:

1. Identify the parts of the bony framework on a diagram of the thorax.
2. Given a diagram, identify the organs that lie within the thoracic cage.
3. Identify and describe the functions of parts of the respiratory system.
4. Define *respiration*.
5. Describe the characteristics of normal respiration.
6. Give normal rates of respiration per minute for various age groups.
7. Describe factors which affect respiration.
8. Discuss the relationship between ventilation and each of the following: metabolic acidosis, respiratory acidosis, metabolic alkalosis, respiratory alkalosis, hypoxia.
9. Identify the normal blood values for pO_2, pCO_2, HCO_3, and pH.

151

TERMINAL OBJECTIVES

Upon completion of this module you are expected to be able to:

1. Define words included in this module's vocabulary.
2. Describe the technique of percussion used in the examination of the thorax and lungs.
3. Describe the technique of auscultation as it is used in the examination of the thorax.
4. Describe the technique of palpation used in the examination of the thorax and lungs.
5. Describe components of inspection of the thorax and lungs.
6. Identify lines of reference and landmarks used in describing locations on the thorax.
7. Identify extrathoracic signs of respiratory disorder.
8. Describe the procedure for evaluation of respiratory excursion.
9. Describe the procedure for evaluation of diaphragmatic excursion.
10. Describe procedures used in evaluating the level of the diaphragm.
11. Name and describe the characteristics of the five major percussion notes.
12. Name and describe the characteristics of the three major breath sounds.
13. Name and describe the characteristics of adventitious sounds.
14. Describe the technique used in evaluating tactile fremitus.
15. Describe techniques used in evaluating vocal resonance (pectoriloquy and egophony).
16. Describe the value of contralateral examination in assessment of thorax and lungs.
17. Describe a screening technique for measuring tidal air volume.
18. Demonstrate inspection, palpation, percussion, and auscultation of the thorax and lungs.
19. Using an assessment form as a guide, take a health history pertinent to the thorax and lungs.
20. Using a physical assessment form as a guide, perform an examination of the thorax and lungs of an adult.
21. Cite features of the examination of the child which differ from those of the adult.
22. Describe biologic changes caused by aging which may affect assessment of the thorax and lungs.
23. Describe variations in physical findings among ethnic groups, if indicated.
24. Record data obtained from the health assessment using appropriate medical terminology.

SUGGESTED ACTIVITIES

Read

Alexander, Mary M., and Marie S. Brown: "The Chest and Lungs," *Pediatric History Taking and Physical Diagnosis for Nurses,* McGraw-Hill, New York, 1979.

Bates, Barbara: "Thorax and Lungs," *A Guide to Physical Examination,* Lippincott, Philadelphia, 1979.

OR

Malasanos, Lois, et al.: "Assessment of the Respiratory System," *Health Assessment,* Mosby, St. Louis, 1977.

Fowkes, William, and Virginia K. Hunn: *Clinical Assessment for the Nurse Practitioner,* Mosby, St. Louis, 1973, p. 61.

Saxon, Sue V., and Mary Jean Etten: *Physical Change and Aging: A Guide for the Helping Professions,* The Tiresias Press, New York, 1978, pp. 90-97.

View

Bates, Barbara: *Examination of the Thorax,* videotape, 6 min.
Physical Assessment of the Heart and Lungs, Program 1: Inspection and Palpation of the Lungs and Thorax, Concept Media filmstrip, 26 min.
Physical Assessment of the Heart and Lungs, Program 2: Percussion and Auscultation of the Lungs and Thorax, Concept Media filmstrip, 50 min.

Equipment

    watercolor felt-tip pen
    gown and drape
    stethoscope having both bell and diaphragm
    centimeter ruler
    centimeter tape

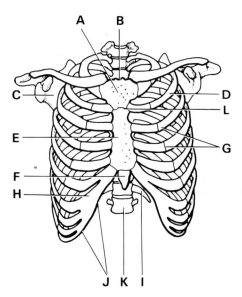

Figure 7-1

PRETEST

1. On Fig. 7-1, identify the parts indicated.

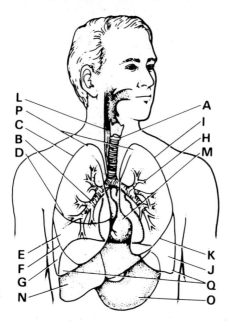

Figure 7-2

2. On Fig. 7-2, label the organs of the thorax as indicated.

3. Indicate the location numbers of the ribs in the following categories:
   a. Vertebrosternal (true) ribs   _____ through _____
   b. Vertebrochondral (false) ribs   _____ through _____
   c. Vertebral (floating) ribs   _____ through_____

4. Match the characteristics or functions in the left column with the organs in the right column.

   _____ Divides into two smaller bronchi

   _____ Serous membrane which covers the diaphragm and surface of the thoracic wall

   _____ Carries blood from the thorax to the superior vena cava

   _____ Divides into seven branches which supply blood to the thorax

   _____ 0.25-mm-wide sacs containing blood capillaries and collageneous, reticular, and elastic tissue fibers in which exchange of gases from air to blood takes place

   _____ Is broad and short, curves slightly, and divides into three smaller bronchi

   _____ 2-cm cylindrical, cartilaginous tube connecting larynx and bronchi

   _____ Serous membrane covering surface of lungs

   _____ Composed of serous, subserous, aerolar, and parenchymal tissue

   _____ Large musculofibrous membrane dividing the thoracic from the abdominal cavity

   a. Trachea
   b. Lungs
   c. Visceral pleura
   d. Parietal pleura
   e. R bronchus
   f. L bronchus
   g. Alveoli
   h. Azygos veins
   i. Diaphragm
   j. Descending aorta

5. Define *respiration.*

6. The correct term used to describe normal breathing is _____ .

7. The ratio of respirations to pulse is _____ to _____ .

8. Give the normal range of respirations per minute for the clients listed below:

   a. Newborn _____

   b. 6-month to 2-year-old _____

   c. Adolescent _____

   d. Adult _____

9. The rate of respirations may be affected by many factors. Name *three* of these.

   a. _____

   b. _____

   c. _____

Write *true* or *false.* If *false,* correct the statement to make it true.

10. _____ The two upper lobes of the lung may be evaluated most easily on the anterior thorax.

11. _____ In expiration, the diaphragm returns to its original position, reducing the pressure in the thoracic cage.

12. _____ The left middle lobe of the lung underlies the left anterior and lateral thorax.

13. _____ The diaphragm may be divided into three portions — sternal, costal, and lumbar.

14. _____ The esophageal hiatus is an opening in the diaphragm through which the esophagus, esophageal blood vessels, and the vagus nerves pass to the abdomen.

15. _____ The vena cava is the vein returning deoxygenated blood to the heart.

16. _____ The respiratory center is located in the stem portion (medulla) of the brain.

17. _____ Alveolar walls are only a single cell in thickness and are composed of squamous epithelium tissue.

18. _____ The 11 intercostales interni extend from cervical vertebrae to outer surfaces of the ribs and increase the size of thoracic cavity.

19. _____ The subcostales muscles attach the upper to the lower ribs and decrease thoracic volume.

20. _____ The xiphoid cartilage may ossify between 30 and 40 years of age.

21. _____ Stimulation of the respiratory center causes an increase in the rate and depth of breathing, thus blowing off excessive CO_2 and increasing the acidity of the blood.

22. _____ The respiratory tract is covered by a protective viscid mucous blanket secreted by goblet and columnar epithelial cells.

23. _____ The hilum of the lung is the point at which the main stem bronchus, pulmonary blood vessels, and nerves join the lungs.

24. _____ A constant positive intrapleural pressure is necessary for normal respirations.

25. _____ The diaphragm is innervated on either side by the vagus nerve.

26. _____ The right main stem bronchus is wider and shorter than the left bronchus.

27. _____ Bronchioles are greater than 1 mm in diameter.

28. _____ Pulmonary surfactant reduces the surface tension of the fluid lining the alveolar epithelium.

29. _____ Sputum is composed of mucus from the tracheobronchial tree, nasal secretions, and salivary gland secretions.

30. _____ Alveolar sacs exist in clusters of 15 to 20 and share common walls between them.

Match definitions in the left column with the terms in the right column.

31. _____ Plasma bicarbonate	a. Tidal volume
32. _____ Volume of air inhaled and exhaled in one breath	b. pO_2
	c. Partial pressure
33. _____ Partial pressure of carbon dioxide in arterial blood	d. Dead space
	e. pH
34. _____ Indication of acid-base balance	f. Residual volume
35. _____ Air in respiratory passageways that is not available for gas exchange	g. HCO_3
	h. Ventilation
36. _____ Partial pressure of oxygen in arterial blood	i. Vital capacity
37. _____ Measure of the total force that a gas exerts against the walls surrounding it	j. pCO_2
37. _____ Process of movement of gas into and out of the pulmonary system	
38. _____ Computed by adding the inspiratory reserve volume, the tidal volume, and the expiratory reserve volume	
39. _____ Gas remaining in the lungs after maximum expiration.	

Match the conditions listed below with the blood gas values shown below in questions 41 to 45.

a. Respiratory acidosis
b. Respiratory alkalosis
c. Metabolic acidosis
d. Metabolic alkalosis
e. Hypoxemia
f. Within normal limits

41. _____ pO_2 70 pCO_2 110 HCO_3 26   pH 7.34
42. _____ pO_2 100 pCO_2 34 HCO_3 34   pH 7.60
43. _____ pO_2 110 pCO_2 35 HCO_3 22   pH 7.43
44. _____ pO_2 45 pCO_2 40 HCO_3 24   pH 7.39
45. _____ pO_2 62 pCO_2 36 HCO_3 30   pH 7.55

VOCABULARY   Descriptive terminology

abdominal respiration
acidosis — metabolic, respiratory
adventitious sounds
alkalosis — metabolic, respiratory
amphoric breathing
anteroposterior thoracic diameter
apnea
arterial blood gases
     pO_2
     pCO_2
     HCO_3
     pH
barrel chest
Biot's breathing
bradypnea
bronchial breathing
bronchophony
bronchovesicular
cellular respiration
cogwheel breath sounds
Cheyne-Stokes respirations
clubbing
dead space
diaphragmatic respirations
dyspnea
egophony
eupnea
expiratory grunts
fremitus
funnel chest

Harrison's groove
hyperpnea
hyperresonance
hyperventilation
Kussmaul's breathing
milk line
orthopnea
paradoxical breathing
partial pressure
pectoriloquy
perfusion
pigeon chest
pleural friction rub
pleximeter
pneumothorax
rales
residual air or volume
resonance
respiration
respiratory excursion
rhonchi
sinus tracts
tachypnea
thoracic respiration
tidal air or volume
ventilation
ventilation-perfusion ratio
vesicular breath sound
vital capacity
wheeze

Diagnostic terminology

acute coryza
adult respiratory distress syndrome
asthma
atelectasis
bronchitis
chronic obstructive pulmonary
  disease (COPD)
emphysema
infant respiratory distress syndrome
influenza

pectus carinatum
pectus excavatum
pleural effusion
pleurisy
pneumonia
pneumothorax
purified protein derivative test (PPD)
pulmonary function tests
tuberculosis

DECISION TABLE 7-1

If . . .		Then . . .
You are having trouble recalling the anatomy and physiology of the thorax and lungs	⟹	Remove and replace organs in torso model.
	⟹	Luckmann, Joan, and Karen Sorensen: *Medical-Surgical Nursing,* Saunders, Philadelphia, 1974, pp. 211-245, 854-857, 870-874.
	⟹	Shapiro, Barry, et al.: *Clinical Application of Respiratory Care,* Year Book, Chicago, 1975, pp. 1-22, 57-89.
	⟹	"Blood-Gas and Acid-Base Concepts in Respiratory Care," *American Journal of Nursing,* 944-963 (June, 1976).
You need a review of the assessment and description of respirations	⟹	Wolff, Luverne, et al.: *Fundamentals of Nursing,* Lippincott, Philadelphia, 1979, pp. 299-303.
	⟹	*Physical Assessment of the Heart and Lungs: Assessing Respirations,* Concept Media filmstrip.
You wish to review the use of the stethoscope	⟹	Littman, David: "Stethoscopes and Auscultation," *American Journal of Nursing,* 1238-1241 (July, 1972).
You love evaluating your progress with programmed-learning modules	⟹	Mechner, Francis, et al.: "Patient Assessment: Examination of the Chest and Lungs," *American Journal of Nursing,* **76**(9):1-22 (September, 1976).
You are interested in additional references pertaining to examination	⟹	Delaney, Mary: "Examining the Chest: The Lungs, Part 1," *Nursing '75,* 12-14 (August, 1975).
	⟹	Jarvis, C. M.: "Performing Physical Assessment," *Nursing '77,* 38-45 (June, 1977).

DECISION TABLE 7-1 (continued)

If . . .		Then . . .
	⟹	Naumoff, Mary Delany: "A Matter of Life and Breath," *Assessing Vital Functions Accurately: Nursing Skillbook,* Nursing '77 Books—Intermed Communications, 1977, pp. 59-68.
You wish to increase your expertise in evaluating breath sounds	⟹	Drugger, Dr. George: *The Chest—Its Sounds and Signs,* Humetrics Corp. audio cassettes (12 cassettes).
You wish additional geriatric information	⟹	Burnside, Irene Mortenson: *Nursing and the Aged,* McGraw-Hill, New York, 1976, pp. 288-290, 297-300.
You are interested in more pediatric references	⟹	Alexander, Mary M., and Marie Scott Brown: "Physical Examination, Part 12: Chest and Lungs," *Nursing '75,* 44-48 (January 1975).
	⟹	Barness, Lewis A.: *Pediatric Physical Diagnosis,* Year Book, Chicago, 1972, pp. 97-110.
You are an advanced student who wants a more complete discussion of respiratory problems of childhood	⟹	Chinn, Peggy L.: *Child Health Maintenance, Concepts in Family Centered Care,* Mosby, St. Louis, 1974, pp. 110-112, 174, 210, 257-268, 315, 350-351.
	⟹	Shapiro, Barry, et al.: *Clinical Application of Respiratory Care,* Year Book, Chicago, 1975, pp. 405-413.
You need to review the relationship between blood gas evaluation and effective functioning of the pulmonary system and to identify signs and symptoms associated with blood gas imbalance	⟹	"Blood-Gas and Acid-Base Concepts in Respiratory Care," *American Journal of Nursing,* 944-963 (June, 1976) (programmed-learning module).
	⟹	Luckmann, Joan, and Karen Sorenson: *Medical-Surgical Nursing, A Psychophysiologic Approach,* Saunders, Philadelphia, 1974, pp. 211-245, 870-874.
	⟹	Oakes, Annalee, and Helen Morrow: "Understanding Blood Gases," *Assessing Vital Functions Accurately: Nursing Skillbook,* Nursing '77 Books—Intermed Communications, 1977, pp. 69-79.
You wish a comprehensive and in-depth look at blood gas physiology (sample patient situations and blood gas problems are given in the appendix along with a discussion of correct answers to problems and rationale for answers)	⟹	Shapiro, Barry A.: *Clinical Application of Blood Gases,* Year Book, Chicago, 1973.

DECISION TABLE 7-1 (continued)

An overview of acid-base balance is desired and programmed learning is the favored method of learning  Cohen, Stephen, et al.: "Metabolic Acid Base Disorders: Part 1," *American Journal of Nursing* (October, 1977); "Part 2: Physiological Abnormalities and Nursing Actions" (January, 1978); "Part 3: Clinical and Laboratory Findings," (March, 1978).

You wish to have an introduction to chest x-rays Tinker, John: "Understanding Chest X-Rays," *American Journal of Nursing,* 54–58 (January, 1976).

POSTTEST

1. At what point would you locate the bases of the lungs at midinspiration?

   a. Anteriorly at the _____ rib

   b. Posteriorly at the _____ rib

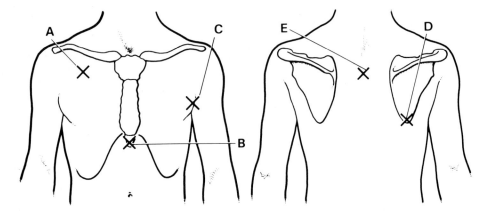

Figure 7-3

2. On Fig. 7-3 identify the location of the abnormalities using appropriate lines of reference and landmarks.

3. Extrathoracic signs of respiratory disease are important in the assessment of the thorax and lungs. Name *five* of these.

   a. _____

   b. _____

   c. _____

    d. _____

    e. _____

4. Cite the principle governing sound vibrations through the chest.

5. All sounds may be evaluated on the basis of *four* characteristics. Name these.

    a. _____

    b. _____

    c. _____

    d. _____

6. Match the percussion notes in the right column with the characteristics describing them in the left column.

_____ Note heard over thigh	a. Resonance
_____ Tone heard over moderately aerated lung	b. Dullness
_____ Drumlike note	c. Flatness
_____ Booming quality typical of emphysema	d. Hyperresonance
_____ Results from moderate increase in density	e. Tympany
_____ Heard over enclosed chambers filled with air	

7. Match the breath sounds in the left column with the characteristic in the right column.

a. Vesicular
b. Bronchovesicular
c. Bronchial
d. Rales
e. Rhonchi
f. Pleural friction rub

_____ Has a blowing, hollow quality and is considered abnormal except over the trachea

_____ May be diagrammed
/\

_____ Caused by lung scraping against pleura

_____ May be heard over trachea

_____ Has a soft, rustling quality

_____ Discrete sounds with a crackling or bubbling quality

_____ May be diagrammed
/\

_____ Heard over major bronchi

_____ Produced by air passing through narrowed bronchi and bronchioles

_____ May be diagrammed
/\

_____ Adventitious sound prominent on expiration and associated with prolonged expiration

Write *true* or *false.* If *false,* correct the statement to make it true.

8. _____ Deeply located masses are best located by percussion.

9. _____ Subcutaneous emphysema is palpated when air leaks from the respiratory tract into subcutaneous tissues.

10. _____ Pigeon chest is noted when there is a deep depression of the sternum which may interfere with cardiac and respiratory function.

11. _____ The angle of Louis is a landmark used to locate the seventh cervical vertebra — the vertebra prominens.

12. _____ Adventitious sounds are variations in normal breath sounds.

13. _____ Breath sounds in children will be more prominent or intense than in adults.

14. _____ Harrison's groove is an abnormal finding in newborn infants.

15. _____ Hyperresonance is a normal sound in a child's lung.

16. _____ One danger to the client during auscultation is that he will hyperventilate.

17. _____ The bell of the stethoscope is usually used in assessing breath sounds.

18. _____ Rales or rhonchi that clear with coughing are most likely not of clinical significance.

19. _____ Most sounds in the lung will be low-pitched; therefore, the diaphragm of the stethoscope should be used for auscultation.

20. _____ Bronchial breath sounds will be heard when pneumothorax has occurred.

21. _____ To "map" an area of abnormally located dullness, one would percuss from the area of dullness to the area of resonance.

22. _____ In percussion of the chest, tones in a specific location of one hemithorax are compared with tones in the comparable location of the opposite hemithorax.

23. _____ Percussion is used to aid in determining density.

24. _____ Tympany would normally be expected in the (R) fifth or sixth intercostal space.

25. _____ Dullness would normally be elicited over the scapulae.

26. _____ The major criterion for evaluating vocal fremitus is that it be of the same intensity over similar areas of both hemithoraces.

27. _____ Vital capacity in an 80-year-old client will be less than in a 20-year-old client.

28. _____ Areas of consolidation must extend to the chest wall for vocal fremitus to be palpated and defined as increased.

29. _____ In egophony, voice sounds are increased in intensity and clarity, and when the patient says "e," it is heard through the stethoscope as "a."

30. _____ In a 1-year-old child a chest circumference greater than the head circumference would be considered abnormal.

31. _____ In examination of an infant, you would expect that extension of the head would accompany inspiration.

32. _____ Breath sounds elicited in a normal infant are bronchovesicular.

33. _____ Fine crepitant rales may be noted at the end of deep inspiration in a normal infant.

34. _____ Breaths taken by an elderly client are not as deep as those taken by a younger client due to a decrease in maximum breathing capacity.

35. _____ An elderly client may present with a complaint of fatigue rather than shortness of breath when suffering an acute respiratory infection.

36. _____ Slight tracheal deviation in an elderly client is a sign of acute respiratory disturbance.

37. _____ Shortness of breath is an indication of an abnormality in a pregnant client during the third trimester.

38. _____ In the elderly client, the vital capacity is increased, leading to a decrease in residual volume, thus decreasing the air available for O_2-CO_2 exchange.

39. _____ Blood gas diffusion is increased in the elderly client.

40. _____ In an infant, seesaw respirations of the lower chest, marked xiphoid retractions, and expiratory grunts audible to the naked ear indicate normal ventilation.

HEALTH HISTORY AND ASSESSMENT

If the answer is yes, place a check (✔)* at the left and provide further information in the Remarks column.

Adult Health History: Thorax and Lungs

Remarks

Do you now have or have you had

_____ Lung or chest disease (example: asthma, pneumonia, tuberculosis, emphysema, cancer)?

Frequency of upper respiratory infections such as colds and flu within last year? _____

_____ Chest surgery?

_____ Chest x-rays, date?_____

_____ A relative or other close associate with tuberculosis?

_____ A positive PPD (TB skin test)?

_____ Pulmonary function tests?

_____ Tracheostomy?

_____ Injury to chest or ribs?

_____ Medications for chest or lung conditions?

_____ Chronic (long-term) exposure to industrial dust, coal dusts, asbestos, etc?

_____ Do you now smoke?

Cigarettes, pipe, cigars, other?_____

Number of cigarettes per day? _____

Length of time smoking?____

_____ A history of smoking?

_____ Coughing?

_____ Cough up sputum or phlegm?

If yes, give color_____

_____ Blood in sputum or phlegm?

_____ Shortness of breath?

*Examiner will obtain further information on all checked items.

_____ Sudden shortness of breath at night?

_____ Pain in chest?

_____ Ache or tightness in chest?

_____ Pain when breathing?

_____ Difficulty taking a deep breath?

_____ Feeling of smothering?

_____ Frequent colds or upper respiratory infections?

_____ Wheezing?

_____ Snoring or noisy breathing?

_____ Dizziness or light-headedness?

_____ Easily tired?

_____ Allergies or hay fever?

_____ Frequent bouts of sneezing?

_____ Frequent hiccups?

_____ Numbness or tingling of fingers, lips, toes?

_____ Blueness of lips, fingers, toes?

_____ Blackout spells?

_____ Bouts of chills and fever?

_____ Night sweats?

_____ Weight loss?

_____ Sleep with more than one pillow?

_____ Edema or swelling?

_____ Bouts of confusion?

_____ Bouts of anxiety for which you cannot account?

Pediatric Adaptations— History

_____ Trouble swallowing?

_____ Inhalation of foreign body?

_____ Measles or infectious disease in last two weeks?

_____ Exposure to recent cold or cough?

_____ Frequent ear infections (otitis media)?

_____ Does child have history of respiratory difficulty (cystic fibrosis, croup, asthma, etc.)?

Number of respiratory infec-

tions in past year _____

Date of PPD _____

Date of DPT _____

Geriatric Adaptations— History

_____ History of emphysema or bronchitis?

_____ Tire easily?

_____ Shortness of breath after mild exertion?

_____ Do you have a cough or wheeze?

Adult Physical Assesment— Thorax and Lungs

Check (✓) if normal, *NE* if not examined, and *X* if abnormal. Describe all abnormal findings.

Description

Describe posture _____

_____ Inspection: No abnormality of chest shape (ratio of AP diameter to lateral diameter between 1 to 2 and 5 to 7)

_____ Thorax is symmetrical in shape and movement

_____ Clavicles not unduly prominent

_____ Scapulae level and same height

_____ Sternum smooth and slightly depressed between hemithoraces

_____ Ribs slope downward at 45° angle

_____ Clearly defined intercostal spaces

_____ Color: No cyanosis of

Skin _____

Lips _____

Nail beds_____

_____ Rapid capillary refilling of nail beds when compressed and released

_____ No clubbing of fingers

_____ Respirations: Man breathing diaphragmatically; woman breathing thoracically, or costally

Rate _____
Inspiration-expiration ratio:

_____

_____ Eupnea

_____ No lag or impairment of respiratory movement

_____ Accessory muscles not used in respiration

_____ No expiratory grunts

_____ No spider nevi

Palpation

_____ Skin warm, smooth, and dry

_____ No masses, lesions, or tenderness

_____ Respiratory excursion equal and symmetrical

_____ No bulging or retraction of interspaces during respiration

_____ No subcutaneous emphysema

_____ Fremitus not increased or decreased

_____ Trachea at midline

_____ Estimated level of diaphragm

Percussion

_____ Diaphragmatic excursion 3 to 5 cm

_____ Dullness over vertebrae and scapulae

_____ Resonance over anterior and posterior lung fields

Auscultation

_____ Voice sounds: Same intensity over both hemithoraces, loudest near airways and decreasing toward periphery

_____ Whispered sounds faint and indistinct

_____ Breath sounds within normal limits:

1. Bronchovesicular over airways
2. Bronchial over trachea
3. Vesicular over remainder of lung

_____ No pleural friction rub

_____ No adventitious sounds

_____ No reduction of vital capacity during match test

Is able to evacuate 95 percent of air from lungs in 3 seconds with forced respirations

Disposition, recommendations, or treatment of abnormal findings:

Pediatric Adaptations— Physical

Description

_____ Chest circumference: _____ cm

_____ Respirations synchronized and symmetrical in upper chest

_____ No retraction of lower chest

_____ Chest contour round

_____ Abdominal breathing prior to age 7

_____ Presence of cough reflex

_____ Diaphragmatic excursion (1 to 2 interspaces)

_____ Breath sounds: Broncho-vesicular

_____ Respirations per minute _____

_____ No paradoxical breathing

_____ No sternal retraction

_____ No expiratory grunts

_____ No audible signs of expiration

_____ No head-rocking with breathing

_____ No flaring of nares

_____ No bouts of cyanosis

_____ No circumoral or periorbital cyanosis

_____ No use of accessory muscles for breathing

If infant, give Apgar score _____

Geriatric Adaptations— Physical

_____ Diminished chest expansion

_____ Reduction of vital capacity with match test

_____ Increase in residual volume (larger lung fields)

Disposition, recommendation, or treatment of abnormal findings:

Student_____

INSTRUCTOR'S GUIDE FOR EVALUATION OF STUDENT PERFORMANCE

Assessment of the thorax and lungs

Behaviors evaluated	Yes	No	Remarks
1. Assembles equipment			
2. Takes appropriate history of the thorax and lungs*			
3. Asks branching questions when indicated*			
4. Explains procedure for examination to client			
5. Washes hands			
6. Gowns and drapes client to prevent undue exposure; removes drape or gown to visualize the entire anterior and posterior chest for symmetry during that portion of exam			
7. Provides quiet environment for examination to aid auscultation			
8. Provides adequate lighting (tangential lighting preferred)			
9. Uses techniques of inspection, palpation, percussion, and auscultation in each phase of examination			
10. Compares hemithoraces in each phase of examination†			
11. Progresses from the neck down in each phase of the examination; the sequence of examination followed is posterior, right and left lateral, and anterior thorax			
12. Correctly evaluates respirations (rate, rhythm, and depth)†			
13. Uses correct technique for inspection			
14. Uses correct technique for palpation			
15. Utilizes correct technique for percussion			
16. Uses correct technique for auscultation			
17. If locating an area of abnormality, defines boundaries by percussing from zones of normal resonance toward the abnormal tone			
18. Avoids scapulae and sternum in auscultation and percussion			

*May be evaluated on the basis of previously submitted history.
†Must correctly perform to pass module.

Behaviors evaluated	Yes	No	Remarks
19. Does not allow the client to hyperventilate during the examination			
20. Records findings using appropriate terminology			
Posterior thorax			
21. Client seated with arms folded across chest for examination			
22. Inspects for symmetry, contour, color, and condition of skin			
23. Palpates posterior interspaces for masses, lesions, etc.			
24. Palpates ribs and scapulae for masses, breaks, etc.			
25. Evaluates tactile fremitus			
26. Evaluates respiratory excursion			
27. Percusses posterior chest in 5-cm intervals from apex to base contralaterally			
28. Using percussion, measures diaphragmatic excursion			
29. Auscultates breath sounds			
30. Auscultates voice and whispered sounds			
Right and left lateral chest			
31. Client seated with arms on head for examination of lateral thoraces			
Lateral thoraces			
32. Begins examination in axillae and proceeds downward contralaterally; uses at least four sites for comparison			
33. Inspects for symmetry in color and condition			
34. Palpates ribs and interspaces for masses and bulges			
35. Palpates for tactile fremitus			
36. Percusses lateral thoraces			
37. Auscultates breath sounds			
38. Auscultates breath and whispered sounds			

Behaviors evaluated	Yes	No	Remarks
Anterior thorax			
39. Client is supine for examination with arms abducted for examination (In examination of child, child is placed totally flat and head isn't allowed to turn.)			
40. Inspects anterior chest for symmetry, contour, color, condition			
41. Palpates ribs and interspaces for bulges and masses			
42. Palpates for tactile fremitus			
43. Palpates trachea			
44. Percusses anterior chest at 5-cm intervals			
45. Auscultates for breath sounds			
46. Auscultates for voice and whispered sounds, if indicated			
47. Performs screening test for obstructive pulmonary disease, if indicated			

Instructor _____ Date _____

MODULE 8

ASSESSMENT OF THE CARDIOVASCULAR SYSTEM

Cardiovascular disease is a leading cause of death in both adults and children; therefore, skill in assessing this system is essential. Early detection of abnormalities can save lives and prevent needless crippling.

This instructional module is designed as a guide to assist you in learning a thorough and systematic approach for obtaining a health history and making an assessment of the cardiovascular system. Emphasis will be on:

1. The normal heart sounds and their physiological basis.
2. The normal cardiac rates and rhythm.
3. The components of and factors affecting blood pressure.
4. The location and importance of peripheral pulses.

The examination techniques which will be used include inspection, palpation, percussion, and auscultation.

The format for this module is similar to that of previous modules. You are to complete this module and pass the Posttest before the scheduled practicum for assessment of the cardiovascular system.

If you have questions, contact your instructor.

PREREQUISITE OBJECTIVES

You should be able to:

1. Label the chambers, vessels, and valves on a diagram of the heart.
2. Differentiate between the structural layers of the pericardium.
3. Trace the circulation of blood through the heart to the left elbow.

175

4. Trace the conduction system of the heart.
5. List and describe the function of the three structures present in fetal circulation which should not be found in adult circulation.
6. On a diagram of the heart, identify the major coronary arteries and the ventricles they supply.
7. Explain the components of blood pressure in relation to the events of the cardiac cycle.
8. List the five factors which influence arterial pressure.

TERMINAL OBJECTIVES

Upon completion of this module you are expected to be able to:

1. On a diagram, label the following areas of the chest: angle of Louis, pulmonic area, aortic area, apical area, tricuspid area, epigastric area, midclavicular area, and midsternal area.
2. Identify the physiological basis for the following heart sounds:
   a. S_1
   b. S_2
   c. S_3
   d. S_4
   e. Opening snap
   f. Ejection click
3. Locate the apical impulse.
4. Identify the location, duration, and size of the PMI.
5. Discuss normal variations affecting the PMI.
6. Identify major areas for precardial inspection and palpation.
7. Demonstrate correct use and placement of the stethoscope.
8. Demonstrate the correct positioning of the client for the auscultation of heart sounds.
9. Identify the location of the peripheral pulses.
10. Demonstrate correct palpation of the peripheral pulses:
    carotid
    radial
    ulnar
    brachial
    femoral
    popliteal
    posterior tibial
    dorsalis pedis
11. Measure jugular venous pressure.
12. State expected changes in the heart rate during pregnancy.

13. Explain the normal physiologic alteration in the heart's position during pregnancy.
14. Describe the altered location of the apical impulse of the heart during pregnancy.
15. Describe the expected changes in heart sounds during pregnancy.
16. State expected changes of the arterial blood pressure during pregnancy.
17. State the factors which contribute to edema.
18. Define *supine hypotension of pregnancy.*

SUGGESTED ACTIVITIES

Read

Alexander, Mary, and Marie Brown: *Pediatric History Taking and Physical Diagnosis for Nurses,* McGraw-Hill, New York, 1979.

Bates, Barbara: *A Guide to Physical Examination,* Lippincott, Philadelphia, 1979 (chapters on the heart and pressures and pulses).
OR
Malasanos, Lois, et al.: *Health Assessment,* Mosby, St. Louis, 1977 (section on cardiovascular assessment).

Caird, F. I., and T. G. Judge, *Assessment of the Elderly Patient,* Pitman, Calif., 1977.
OR
Saxon, Sue V., and Mary Jean Etten: *Physical Change and Aging,* The Tiresias Press, New York, 1978.

Ziegel, Erna, and Mecca Cranley: "Maternal Physiologic Changes During Pregnancy," *Obstetric Nursing,* Macmillan, New York, (on changes in the cardiovascular system).
OR
Jensen, Margaret Duncan, et al.: "Maternal Physiology — Cardiovascular Changes," *Maternity Care: The Nurse and the Family,* Mosby, St. Louis,

View

Physical Assessment: Heart and Lungs, Program 5, Initial Assessment of the Heart, Concept Media Video casssette.
Physical Assessment: Heart and Lungs, Program 6, Auscultation of the Heart, Concept Media video cassette.
Ravin, Abe: *Cardiac Auscultation,* Merck, Sharp, and Dome audio cassettes.
Bates, Barbara: *Visual Guide to Physical Examination — Peripheral Vascular System,* Lippincott video cassette.
_____: *Visual Guide to Physical Examination — Heart,* Lippincott video cassette.
Pediatric Examination — The Cardiovascular System, Blue Hill Series videotape.
Physical Assessment — Cardiovascular, Blue Hill Series videotape.

Equipment

cape or gown
stethoscope with bell and diaphragm
sphygmomanometer

PRETEST   1. Label the chambers, vessels, and valves of the heart in Fig. 8-1.

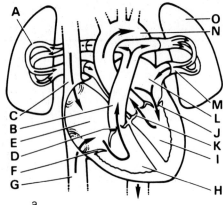

Figure 8-1

a.

b.

c.

d.

e.

f.

g.

h.

i.

j.

k.

l.

m.

n.

o.

2. Beginning with the lungs, name the anatomical structures through which oxygenated blood passes on its way to the left elbow.

a.

b.

c.

d.

e.

f.

g.

3. List *five* factors which influence arterial pressure.

a. _____

b. _____

c. _____

    d. _____

    e. _____

4. The diastolic blood pressure measures _____.

5. Draw a diagram of the heart showing its conduction system.

6. The myocardium is the (*inside, middle, outside*) layer of muscle in the heart.

7. Name and describe the functions of the *three* structures present in fetal circulation which are not normally found in adult circulation.

    a. _____

    b. _____

    c. _____

VOCABULARY

aneurysm	ejection click	PMI
angina	endocardium	precordial bulge
angle of Louis	epicardium	precordium
aortic murmur	functional murmur	S_1
apical impulse	gallop	S_2
arrhythmia	hepatomegaly	S_3
atrium	holosystolic	S_4
bradycardia	hyperemia	semilunar valve
clubbing	hypertension	split sound
cyanosis	hypotension	superior vena cava
central	inferior vena cava	systole
peripheral	mitral regurgitation	tachycardia
diastole	mitral valve	thrill
diastolic murmur	myocardium	tricuspid valve
dyspnea	orthopnea	varicosities
ectopic	pallor	venous stasis
edema	palpitation	ventricle
localized	pericardial rub	
dependent	pericardium	
generalized	petechiae	
pitting	phlebitis	

DECISION TABLE 8-1

If . . .		Then . . .
You need more help with the general anatomy and physiology of the cardiovascular system	⟹	*Anatomy of the Heart,* Merck, Sharpe, Dome videotape (2).
You need help with fetal circulation and pediatric cardiac anatomy and physiology	⟹	*Fetal Circulation and Adult Circulation,* CIBA slides.
You need help with blood pressure	⟹	American Heart Association: *Blood Pressure* (pamphlet).
You need help in taking a complete history	⟹	American Heart Association: *Examination of the Heart: Part 1, Data Collection: The Clinical History* (booklet).
You need help in palpating the chest	⟹	American Heart Association: *Examination of the Heart, Part 3, Inspection and Palpation of the Anterior Chest* (booklet).
You need help in auscultation of heart sounds	⟹	*Interpreting Heart Sounds,* Hoffman-LaRoche, audio cassette, booklet, and self-examination quiz, 1972.
	⟹	Diamond, E. Gary: *Heart Sounds and Auscultation: A Heart Sound Tape for Physicians, Nurses, and Medical Students,* American College of Cardology, audio cassette and text, 1973, 50 min.
You need help in interpreting ECG patterns	⟹	Dale, Dubin: *Rapid Interpretation of ECG's,* Cover Publishing Co., Tampa, Fla., 1974 (programmed text).
	⟹	American Heart Association: *Examination of the Heart, Part 5: The Electrocardiogram* (booklet).
You need help with assessment of pediatric murmurs	⟹	Guntheroth, Warren G., "Initial Evaluation of the Child for Heart Disease," *Pediatric Clinics of North America,* 661–665 (November, 1978).

POSTTEST

1. Label Fig. 8-2 with the areas of the chest.

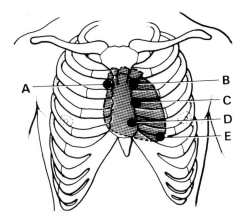

Figure 8-2

a.

b.

c.

d.

e.

2. The heart is assessed primarily through the (*anterior, posterior*) chest wall.

3. The left ventricle is clinically important because it forms the left border and pro-duces the _____.

4. The apical impulse is usually found in the _____ interspace at the _____ line.

5. During pregnancy the apical impulse is rotated _____ and _____.
   a. Leftward
   b. Rightward
   c. Upward
   d. Downward

6. Normal heart sounds are produced by _____.

7. Trace the conduction system of the heart.

8. The SA nodes function as a _____.

9. S_1 heart sound is produced by the closure of the _____.

10. S_2 heart sound is produced by the closure of the _____.

11. S_1 is best heard at the _____ of the heart.

12. S_2 is best heard at the _____ of the heart.

13. S_3 heart sound is produced by the _____.

14. S_3 is a normal sound in _____.

15. S_4 heart sound is produced by _____.

16. The opening snap, (OS), normally a silent event, may be heard in _____

_____.

Write *true* or *false.* If *false,* correct the statement to make it true.

17. _____ Tangential lighting helps to detect pulsations.

18. _____ The tips of the fingers are most sensitive for detecting heart thrills.

19. When an irregularity in the heart rate is auscultated, the rate should be counted for at least _____.

20. The anatomical landmarks of the location of murmurs should be described in terms of _____ and _____ from the midsternal or midclavicular lines.

21. Name *five* signs and symptoms of cardiovascular disease which may be identified from inspection of the client.

a. _____

b. _____

c. _____

d. _____

e. _____

22. The bell of the stethoscope is used to listen for _____.

23. Venous pressure is (*lower, higher*) than arterial pressure.

24. Venous pressure is a measurement of

   a. _____

   b. _____

   c. _____

25. Venous pressure can be measured by inspection of the _____ vein.

26. Venous pressure, measured by inspection and palpation, is estimated from the

   _____   _____ .

27. Pressures more than _____ above the sternal angles are considered elevated.

28. Central venous pressures, which provides information about the degree of cardiac compensation, can be estimated from the _____.

29. Name *four* pulses that should be palpated in the lower extremities.

   a. _____

   b. _____

   c. _____

   d. _____

Write *true* or *false.* If *false,* correct the statement to make it true.

30. _____ The heart rate may normally increase as much as 15 beats per minute over nonpregnant levels during pregnancy.

31. _____ The heart is pushed to the left posterior aspect of the chest cavity during pregnancy.

32. _____ The apical pulse of the woman advanced in pregnancy may be located higher than in the nonpregnant woman.

33. _____ Diastolic murmurs are common throughout pregnancy due to increased blood volume and increased cardiac output.

34. _____ Arterial blood pressure rises normally throughout pregnancy.

35. _____ Dependent leg edema may be considered normal in pregnancy.

36. _____ Supine hypotension in pregnancy is a common phenomenon.

37. _____ Palpitations of the heart are a normal occurrence in pregnancy.

38. _____ The normal PMI in an infant is the sixth intercostal space lateral to the midclavicular line.

HEALTH HISTORY AND ASSESSMENT

Adult Health History: Cardiovascular System

If the answer is yes, place a check (✔) at the left and provide further information in the Remarks column.

Remarks

_____ Worried about your heart?

_____ Ever been told your blood pressure was too high or too low?

_____ Pains in heart or chest?

_____ Heart pounding or skipping a beat?

_____ Heart starts racing suddenly?

_____ Ever told you had a murmur?

_____ Any shortness of breath?

_____ Require more than one pillow for sleeping?

_____ Sudden shortness of breath at night?

_____ Coughing up sputum?

_____ Ever cough up blood-tinged sputum?

_____ Swelling of ankles?

_____ Urination during night?
　　How many times?_____

_____ Dizziness or fainting?

_____ Numbness or tingling of arms or legs?

_____ Leg cramps in bed or sitting still?

_____ Leg cramps while walking?

_____ Previous ECG?
　　Date? _____

_____ Taking medicine for heart?
　　What? _____

_____ Taking medicine for blood pressure?
　　What? _____

_____ Blood type? _____

_____ Have you ever had a blood transfusion?
　　If yes, amount, when, why?
　　Reaction? _____

_____ Have you ever been told you were anemic?

_____ Taking iron pills?

_____ Exercise daily?

Type? _____

_____ How do you release stress?

_____

_____ How do you relax?

_____

_____ Ever been told you had:

    _____ Stroke?

    _____ Vein trouble?

    Hardening of the arteries (atherosclerosis)?

    _____ High cholesterol or fat levels in your blood (hyperlipidemia)?

    _____ To reduce your salt intake?

    _____ Rheumatic fever?

    _____ A bleeding tendency?

_____ Family history of heart trouble?

_____ Family history of congenital heart defects?

_____ Smoke? Number of cigarettes or other tobacco per day?

_____

_____ Number of alcoholic drinks per

day?_____

    What kind? _____

_____ Hours of sleep per night? _____

Pediatric Adaptations— History

_____ Apgar scores?

1 min _____

5 min _____

_____ Circumoral cyanosis/duskiness as newborn?

_____ Quality of suck?

_____ Tires easily (especially during feeding for infants)?

_____ Appetite poor, anorexia?

_____ Vomits frequently?

_____ Color changes during feeding?

_____ Darkening of color when crying?

_____ Weight loss or poor weight gain?

_____ Edema of eyelids?

_____ Squats frequently, especially while playing?

_____ Sleeps in knee-to-chest position beyond 2 years?

_____ Shortness of breath relieved by squatting or sitting up?

_____ Bloody, frothy sputum?

_____ Persistent hacking cough?

_____ Tolerates exercise well?

_____ Frequent chest colds?

_____ Takes infections easily?

_____ Amount of fluids taken per day?

_____ Amount of iron intake per day?

_____ Maternal history

    _____ Amount of alcohol consumed per day during pregnancy?

    _____

    _____ Infections during pregnancy? _____

    _____ Medications taken during pregnancy? _____

        Prescription _____

        Nonprescption _____

_____ Migratory joint pain?

_____ Jerking episodes (chorea)?

_____ Epistaxis?

_____ Rashes?

_____ Abdominal pain?

_____ Fever?

_____ Substernal pain that subsides
with rest?

_____ List all medications taken by
child

Prescription_____

_____

Nonprescription_____

_____

**Geriatric
Adaptations—
History**

_____ Tire easily?

_____ Shortness of breath?

_____ After walking a block
on even surface?

_____ After walking up a
flight of stairs?

_____ After going to bed?

_____ Exercise regularly?

Type of exercise _____

How often _____

_____ Chest pain?

_____ History of heart disease?

_____ Any dizziness when sitting or
standing?

_____ Varicose veins?

**Adult Physical
Assessment—
Cardiovascular
System**

Check (✔) if normal, _NE_ if not examined, and _X_ if abnormal. Describe all abnormal
findings.

Heart   Description

_____ PMI left midclavicular line

_____ Chest symmetrical

_____ No thrills palpated

_____ Regular sinus rhythm, rate:

_____

_____ Aortic-pulmonic S_2 is greater
than S_1, no murmurs, rubs

_____ Tricuspid-mitral: S_1 is greater than S_2, no murmurs, rubs, no S_3 or S_4

_____ Jugular venous pressure is less than 3 cm above sternal angle

_____ Carotid pulses 4+ and symmetrical

Peripheral vascular

_____ Arms and hands: Skin and nail beds pink, smooth, warm, and dry

_____ No clubbing

_____ Radial, ulnar, and brachial pulses 4+ (on 0 to 4 scale)

_____ Epitrochlear nodes: Nonpalpable, nontender

_____ Legs and feet: Skin and nail beds pink, smooth, warm, and dry

_____ No pretibial, ankle, or hand edema

_____ No varicosities, ulceration

_____ Homans's sign negative, no calf tenderness

_____ Femoral, popliteal, posterior tibial, and dorsalis pedis pulses 4+ (on 0 to 4 scale)

_____ Inguinal nodes: Nonpalpable, nontender

Pediatric Adaptations— Physical

_____ No acrocyanosis

_____ No pallor or cyanosis of oral mucosa

_____ No hepatomegaly

_____ No precordial bulge

_____ Chest symmetrical, no left parasternal bulge

_____ PMI fourth intercostal space left MCL

_____ No visible suprasternal pulsations

_____ Normal weight gain and body size

_____ Leg and arm diastolic pressure equal

_____ Pulse pressure between 20 and 50 mm Hg

_____ No tachycardia (above 160 in sleeping NB)

_____ No tachypnea (consistently above 60 in sleeping NB)

_____ No paroxysmal hyperpnea

_____ No rapid, shallow respirations

_____ No rales

_____ No wheezing

_____ No decreased vital and total lung capacity

_____ No abdominal pain

_____ No diaphoresis or cold sweat on forehead

_____ No persistent heat rash

_____ No subcutaneous nodules

Geriatric Adaptations— Physical

_____ Blood pressure in both arms lying and sitting are within normal limits for age

_____ Equal, full brachial, femoral, and carotid pulses

_____ No cyanosis

_____ Extremities warm

Recommendations, treatment, or disposition of abnormal findings:

Student_____

INSTRUCTOR'S GUIDE FOR EVALUATION OF STUDENT PERFOR- MANCE

Assessment of the Cardiovascular System

Behaviors evaluated	Yes	No	Remarks
1. Assembles equipment			
2. Explains procedure to client			
3. Positions client in supine position or upper body elevated 30 to 45°			
4. Assures quiet environment			
5. Proceeds in orderly fashion to *inspect:*			
a. The aortic area			
b. The pulmonary area			
c. The right ventricular area			
d. The left ventricular area			
e. The epigastric area			
6. Proceeds in orderly fashion to *percuss* border of cardiac dullness			
7. Proceeds in orderly fashion to *auscultate* heart sounds, rate, and rhythm in the following locations:			
(1) Aortic area			
(2) Pulmonic area			
(3) Third left interspace			
(4) Tricuspid area			
(5) Mitral area			
8. Uses diaphragm of stethopscope first for identifying high-pitched sounds (S_1, S_2)			
9. Uses bell of stethoscope for identifying low-pitched sounds (S_3, S_4)			
10. Explores surrounding chest surface for distribution of abnormal sounds			
11. Uses special positions to elicit or accentuate abnormalities			
12. Describes abnormalities in terms of			
a. Timing in relation to cardiac cycle			
b. Their location			

Behaviors evaluated	Yes	No	Remarks
Examination of arterial pulse			
13. Examines radial artery with pads of index and middle finger			
14. Examines carotid artery one side at a time			
15. Describes rate and rhythm of pulse			
16. Describes amplitude of pulse			
17. Describes contour of pulse			
18. Examines jugular vein:			
a. Positions patient comfortably with head slightly elevated			
b. Identifies highest point at which pulsations of internal jugular vein are visible			
c. Measures vertical distance between this point and sternal angle			
d. Records distance in centimeters above sternal angle together with angle at which patient is lying			
e. Observes amplitude and timing of jugular venous pulsations			
19. Examines peripheral pulses:			
a. Radial			
b. Ulnar			
c. Brachial			
d. Femoral			
e. Popliteal			
f. Posterior tibial			
g. Dorsalis pedis			

Instructor _____ Date _____

MODULE 9

ASSESSMENT OF THE ABDOMEN, PART 1

This instructional module is designed as a guide to assist you in learning a thorough and systematic approach for assessment of the abdomen. Emphasis is placed on taking an appropriate health history and learning inspection, palpation, percussion, and auscultation of the abdomen. Adaptations for assessing the infant, child, and geriatric client are included in this module. Abdominal assessment of the geriatric client is similar to assessment of the adult. Assessment of the pregnant, intrapartal, and postpartal abdomen is included in Module 10.

The format for this module is similar to the previous modules. You are to complete the material and pass the Posttest before the scheduled laboratory period for assessment of the abdomen.

If you have difficulty in completing the module, contact your instructor.

PREREQUISITE OBJECTIVES   You should be able to:

1. Label the four quadrants and the periumbilical, epigastric, and suprapubic regions on a diagram of the abdomen.
2. On a diagram of the abdomen or a torso model, name and give the location of the major abdominal organs.
3. Describe the functions of the liver, pancreas, spleen, and gallbladder.

4. Describe the digestive processes that occur in the stomach, small intestine, and large intestine.
5. Discuss the effect of the autonomic nervous system on peristalsis.

TERMINAL OBJECTIVES

Upon completion of this module you are expected to be able to:

1. Define the vocabulary words accompanying this module.
2. Given an assessment form as a guide, take a health history pertinent to the abdomen and digestive system using appropriate branching questions.
3. Perform an abdominal examination on an adult, using an assessment form as a guide.
4. Record the data obtained from the health assessment using correct medical terminology.
5. List eight observations to be made during inspection of the abdomen.
6. Describe the areas of auscultation of the abdomen.
7. Describe the sounds of bruits and bowel sounds.
8. Name the five percussion notes and give an example of each.
9. Demonstrate percussion of the liver, spleen, and gastric air bubble.
10. Demonstrate light and deep palpation of the abdomen.
11. Demonstrate palpation for rebound tenderness and costovertebral angle (CVA) tenderness.
12. Demonstrate palpation of the liver, spleen, kidneys, and aorta.
13. Using the OMNI palpation blocks or other simulated material, describe the surface characteristics, consistency, shape, size, and mobility of the simulated structures.
14. Approximate the size in centimeters of given figures without the use of a centimeter ruler.
15. Describe the anatomical differences existing between the child and the adult that will be of significance to the examiner.
16. Describe approaches to the child which will aid the nurse in preparing and positioning the child for examination.
17. Describe techniques used in examination of the child.
18. Describe biologic changes in the digestive system due to aging which should be considered in assessing the health of the geriatric client.
19. Describe variations in physical findings among ethnic groups.

SUGGESTED ACTIVITIES

Read

Alexander, Mary, and Marie Brown: "Abdomen," *Pediatric History Taking and Physical Diagnosis for Nurses,* McGraw-Hill, New York, 1979.

Bates, Barbara: "Abdomen, Adult and Child," *A Guide to Physical Examination,* Lippincott, Philadelphia, 1974.

OR

Malasanos, Lois, et al.: "Abdomen," *Health Assessment,* Mosby, St. Louis, 1977.

Caird, F. I., and T. G. Judge: "Gastrointestinal System," *Assessment of the Elderly Patient,* Pitman, Calif., 1977.

OR

Saxon, Sue V., and Mary Jean Etten: "The Digestive System," *Physical Change and Aging,* The Tiresias Press, New York, 1978.

View

Bates, Barbara: *Examination of the Abdomen,* Lippincott videotape, 9 min.

OR

Physical Assessment Examinations: The Abdomen, Blue-Hill Educational Systems videotape, 35 min.

Biologic Changes of Aging: Function and Capacity, Digestive System, Trainex program 454, slides 43-51.

Pediatric Physical Examination, Abdomen and Genitalia, Blue-Hill Educational Systems videotape, 44 min.

Touchy-Feely, OMNI Education, tactile palpation blocks.

Equipment

marking pen
stethoscope
centimeter ruler
gown
drape
Lange or Harpenden calipers
anthrogauge (if desired)
measuring tape, 7 to 12 mm wide

PRETEST   With books closed, test your knowledge of anatomy and physiology of the abdomen.

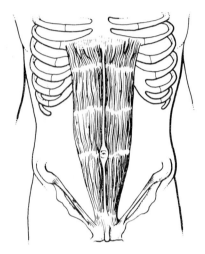

Figure 9-1

1. Using Fig. 9-1, draw and label the four abdominal quadrants.
2. On Fig. 9-1, label the following areas: suprapubic, periumbilical, epigastric.
3. On Fig. 9-1, indicate the correct location for each of the following organs:

   a. Liver
   b. Stomach
   c. Spleen
   d. Kidney
   e. Ovaries and tubes
   f. Uterus

   g. Gallbladder
   h. Bladder
   i. Hepatic flexure
   j. Splenic flexure
   k. Cecum
   l. Duodenum

4. The nerve fibers that stimulate peristalsis are the

   a. Sympathetic nervous system
   b. Parasympathetic nervous system
   c. Central nervous system

5. List *four* functions of the liver.

   a. _____

   b. _____

   c. _____

   d. _____

6. List *two* functions of the gallbladder.

   a. _____

   b. _____

7. State *one* major function of bile. _____

_____

8. The bile pigment that results from the decomposition of hemoglobin is called

_____. An increase in the amount

of this pigment in the blood causes the symptom of _____.

VOCABULARY

Descriptive terminology

anorexia	diastasis recti	hernia
ascites	dysphagia	jaundice
borborygmus	epigastrium	organomegaly
bruits	flatulence	splenomegaly
costovertebral angle (CVA)	hepatomegaly	striae

Diagnostic terminology

aneurysm	cirrhosis	paralytic ileus	pylorospasm
cholecystitis	diverticulitis	peritonitis	varices

DECISION TABLE 9-1

If . . .		Then . . .
You prefer programmed instruction	⟹	Mansell, E: "Patient Assessment of the Abdomen," *American Journal of Nursing,* **74**(2), (1974).
You prefer well-illustrated material	⟹	A. H. Robins Co., *G. I. Series: Physical Examination of the Abdomen* (booklet).
You desire an additional geriatric reference that discusses nutritional needs and digestive disorders of the aged	⟹	Burnside, Irene M.: *Nursing and the Aged,* McGraw-Hill, New York, 1976.
You need help with history taking and branching questions pertinent to the gastrointestinal tract	⟹	Wasson, John, et al.: *The Common Symptom Guide,* McGraw-Hill, New York, 1975 (abdominal pain, blood in stools, vomiting blood).
You want more information on pediatric nutritional assessment	⟹	Zerfas, Alfred J.: "Office Assessment of Nutritional Status," *Pediatric Clinics of North American,* 253-272 (February, 1977).
	⟹	Pipes, Peggy I.: *Nutrition in Infancy and Childhood,* Mosby, St. Louis, 1977.

DECISION TABLE 9-1 (continued)

If. . .		Then. . .
You want more tables for arm circumference and skin-fold norms	⟹	Frisancho, A. Roberto: "Triceps Skin Fold and Upper Arm Muscle Size Assessment of Nutritional Status," *American Journal of Clinical Nutrition*, **27**:1052–1058 (October, 1974).
You want information about common errors in pediatric measurements	⟹	Zerfas, Alfred J.: "Office Assessment of Nutritional Status," *Pediatric Clinics of North America*, 259 (February, 1977).

POSTTEST

1. List *six* major symptoms to be assessed in the gastrointestinal history.

   a. _____

   b. _____

   c. _____

   d. _____

   e. _____

   f. _____

2. The history of a recent increase in appetite that is not associated with a weight gain is a significant diagnostic finding. Name *one* clinical example.

   _____

3. List *four* characteristics of any excretion (e.g., vomitus or drainage) that should be ascertained and recorded:

   a. _____

   b. _____

   c. _____

   d. _____

4. List *three* changes in the stomach or intestine that are due to aging.

   a. _____

   b. _____

   c. _____

5. Dysphagia in a geriatric client that is associated with slowness in eating, choking, and sputtering is probably

   a. Neurological in origin

   b. Due to an obstruction of the esophagus

   c. Due to muscle weakness, a part of the normal aging process

6. The stomach is located in the
   a. Right upper quadrant
   b. Left upper quadrant
   c. Epigastrium
7. The normal size of the adult liver in the right midclavicular line is approximately
   a. 4 to 8 cm
   b. 6 to 12 cm
   c. 10 to 16 cm
   d. 14 to 18 cm
8. Tenderness of the posterior costovertebral angle is most commonly due to pathology of the
   a. Liver
   b. Spleen
   c. Kidney
   d. Vertebral disk
9. Rebound tenderness is indicative of
   a. Liver enlargement
   b. Bladder distention
   c. Kidney infection
   d. Peritonitis

Write *true* or *false.*

10. _____ The adult spleen is generally palpable when it is twice the normal size.
11. _____ Both adult kidneys are usually palpable.

12. *Two* purposes of deep palpation are to determine:

   a. _____

   b. _____

13. Number the correct sequence for assessing the abdomen.
   _____ Inspection
   _____ Palpation
   _____ Percussion
   _____ Auscultation

14. Match the following percussion notes. The notes may be used more than once.

   a. _____ Distended bladder
   b. _____ Gastric air bubble
   c. _____ Liver
   d. _____ Gas in colon

   1. Flatness
   2. Dullness
   3. Resonance
   4. Hyperresonance
   5. Tympany

15. The frequency of bowel sounds is approximately _____ to
_____ per minute.

16. Bowel sounds are considered hyperactive when auscultation reveals
    a. 1, 2   1. Increased frequency and intensity of sounds
    b. 3, 4   2. Loud and continuous sounds
    c. 1, 2, 3   3. Loud, high-pitched, metallic tinkling sound alternating
    d. All of these   with periods of silence
                     4. High-pitched, soft and gurgling sounds

Write *true* or *false*.

17. _____ An elderly person with large lung fields may have a normal liver that is palpable 1 to 2 cm below the right costal margin.

18. _____ The elderly person rarely exhibits a rigid abdomen as a manifestation of peritoneal irritation.

19. Is diastasis recti a *normal* or *abnormal* finding in children? _____

20. List *three* approaches that may be taken by the examiner to aid in preparing the child for an abdominal examination.

    a. _____

    b. _____

    c. _____

21. List *three* characteristics that should be noted in evaluation of an umbilical hernia of the child.

    a. _____

    b. _____

    c. _____

22. If upon examination of the abdomen of the child visible peristalic waves proceeding from left to right are noted, would you consider this finding *normal* or *abnormal?* _____

23. Examination of a 14-month-old child reveals enlargement of the liver which is palpable 1.5 cm below the right costal margin. Is this finding *normal* or *abnormal?*

    _____

24. The normal child's abdomen may best be described as having _____ appearance.

25. Are distended veins visible on the abdomen considered *normal* or *abnormal?*

    _____

26. With the exception of liver dullness, percussion notes over the remainder of the abdomen of a child may be described as _____.

27. Inspection of the umbilicus of the neonate for signs of abnormality or infection is a prime responsibility of the nurse. List *three* findings which would alert the nurse to the presence of abnormality.

    a. _____

    b. _____

    c. _____

28. Describe techniques for eliciting the location of tenderness and a description of pain when examining the child.

29. Deep palpation of the midepigastrium of the child causes him to wince and complain of pain. Is this finding *normal* or *abnormal?* Explain.

30. Normal kidneys are often difficult to palpate in the child. The portion palpated by the examiner will be the _____.

31. The cecum in the child will present a soft, gas-filled object in the_____ quadrant of the abdomen; the sigmoid, as a freely moveable sausage-shaped mass in the _____ quadrant.

32. In your examination of a 6-month-old infant, you note that respiration occurs primarily by abdominal breathing. Is this *normal* or *abnormal?*

HEALTH HISTORY AND ASSESSMENT

Adult Gastro-intestinal History

If the answer is yes, place a check (✔) at the left and provide further information in the Remarks column.

Remarks

Description of typical daily meal plan

_____ Snacking? What?

_____ Special likes?

_____ Special dislikes?

_____ Foods that disagree? What?

_____ Medical restrictions on diet?

_____ Religious restrictions on diet?

_____ Impaired ability to feed self?

_____ Mechanical difficulty in chewing food?

_____ How much fluid consumed in a day?_____What?_____

_____ Poor appetite?

_____ Nausea or vomiting?

_____ Vomiting of blood?

_____ Indigestion, heartburn, or food intolerance?

_____ Belching, gas?

_____ Yellow skin or eyes?

_____ Burning or hunger pains in stomach?

_____ Difficulty in swallowing?

_____ Soreness, pain, or cramps in abdomen?

_____ Diarrhea?

_____ Constipation?

_____ Black or tarry stools?

_____ Mucus in stools?

_____ Use laxatives or enemas frequently?

_____ Recent change in bowel habits?

_____ Rectal bleeding or pain?

_____ Family history of colitis, ulcers, or enteritis?

Drugs taken: _____

Adult Physical Check (✔) if normal, *NE* if not examined, *X* if abnormal. Describe abnormal findings.

Description

_____ Skin: No scars, striae, rashes, lesions, or dilated veins

_____ Umbilicus: Normal contour, no

herniation, contour _____

_____ No distention, rigidity, or ascites

_____ Liver size within 6 to 12 cm midclavicular

_____ Bowel sounds present, no hyperactivity

_____ No bruits or friction rubs

_____ Light palpation: No masses or tenderness

_____ Deep palpation: No masses or tenderness, or rebound tenderness

_____ Liver, spleen, kidneys non-palpable, nontender

_____ No CVA tenderness

_____ Inguinal lymph nodes: Non-palpable, nontender

_____ No inguinal or femoral herniation

Geriatric Adaptations— History

Remarks

_____ Alternating constipation and diarrhea?

_____ Intolerance of fatty foods?

_____ Heartburn, belching, or chest pain when lying down after a meal?

_____ Abdominal pain?

    _____ Associated with vomiting?

    _____ Related to food?

    _____ Relieved by defecation?

_____ Difficulty in swallowing solids? liquids?

Physical   Description

_____ Normal aorta width 2.5 to 4 cm

_____ No liver enlargement (liver may be 1 to 2 cm below right costal margin due to large lung fields)

_____ No fecal impaction

Pediatric Adaptations— History

_____ Number of meals eaten per day?   Remarks

_____ Snacking habits?

_____ Method of feeding?

_____ Eating patterns during illness?

_____ Likes, dislikes?

_____ 24-hour intake sample? List.

_____ Cooking facilities?

_____ Use federal programs (lunch, food stamps, etc.)?

_____ Infant formula

    _____ Type, amount?

    _____ Preparation

_____ Breast-fed infants

    _____ Length of suck at each breast, frequency?

    _____ Weight before and after feeding if equipment is available or infant has poor weight gain?

_____ Mother's diet?

_____ Maternal medications?

    _____ Prescription

    _____ Nonprescription

_____ Maternal habits

    _____ Amount of alcohol per day?

    _____ Number of cigarettes per day?

_____ When were solid foods introduced?

_____ Type of solid food and method of introduction?

_____ Age of weaning?

_____ Amount, quality, consistency, color, frequency of stools?

_____ Amount of milk taken per 24 hours?

_____ Must child eat everything on plate?

_____ Colic?

_____ Draws knees up and cries?

Pediatric Adaptation— Physical

Remarks

_____ Two umbilical arteries and one umbilical vein in cord (neonate)

_____ Cord well healed, no granulomatous tissue (infant)

_____ Umbilical hernia less than 2 to 5 cm (newborn)

_____ No umbilical hernias (beyond 16 months)

_____ No epigastric hernias

_____ No diastasis recti

_____ Liver palpable 1 to 2 cm below right costal margin

_____ Spleen palpable 1 to 2 cm below left costal margin

_____ No visible peristaltic waves

_____ Abdominal respirations present (to age 7)

_____ No scaphoid, flat abdomen (newborn)

Nutritional assessment*

_____ Height/length

_____ Weight

_____ Mid-upper arm circumference

_____ Triceps skin-fold measurement

_____ Head circumference

_____ No apathy

_____ No irritability

_____ No pallor (skin, tongue, mucous membranes, or conjunctival)

_____ No edema

_____ No emaciation

_____ No obesity

_____ No frog-leg position

_____ No nasolabial seborrhea

_____ No dermatitis (perineal, symmetrical, or "crazy pavement")

_____ No follicular hyperkeratosis

_____ No change in hair texture, color, or amount of hair loss

_____ No circumcorneal injection

_____ No gingivitis

_____ No pain, redness, smoothness, atrophy, denudement, or edema of tongue

_____ No parotid enlargement

_____ No craniotabes or cranial bossing

_____ No costochondral beads

_____ No wrist or epiphyseal enlargement

_____ No loss DTR, or vibratory sense

_____ No calf tenderness

Treatment, disposition, and recommendations regarding abnormal findings:

*Adapted from Alfred J. Zerfas, et al., "Office Assessment of Nutritional Status," *Pediatric Clinics of North America,* 253-272 (February, 1977).

Student_____

INSTRUCTOR'S GUIDE FOR EVALUATION OF STUDENT PERFOR- MANCE

Assessment of the Abdomen

Behaviors evaluated	Yes	No	Remarks
1. Assembles equipment needed			
2. Takes appropriate gastrointestinal history*			
3. Asks branching questions as appropriate*			
4. Explains procedure for examination of client			
5. Places client in supine position, knees slightly flexed			
6. Drapes to expose abdomen, keeping other areas covered			
7. Stands at right side of client to perform exam			
8. Inspects abdomen before proceeding			
9. Warms stethoscope by rubbing on palms			
10. Uses diaphragm of stethoscope for auscultation, with ear pieces placed correctly			
11. Listens for bowel sounds in all four quadrants			
12. Listens for bruits over aorta, renal arteries, and iliac vessels			
13. Auscultates before percussing abdomen			
14. Percusses in all four quadrants			
15. Uses correct technique for percussion			
16. Percusses and measures liver			
17. Percusses spleen and gastric air bubble			
18. Percusses before palpating abdomen			
19. Nails of examining hand are short and rounded			
20. Light palpation of all four quadrants			
21. Deep palpation of all four quadrants			
22. Palpates for liver, spleen, kidneys, and aorta			
23. Palpates for rebound tenderness			
24. Palpates for CVA tenderness			
25. Records findings, using appropriate terminology			

*Evaluated on previously submitted history.

Instructor _____ Date _____

MODULE 10

ASSESSMENT OF THE ABDOMEN, PART 2, ADAPTATIONS FOR THE OBSTETRICAL CLIENT

This instructional module is designed as a guide to assist you in learning a thorough and systematic approach for obtaining a health history and making an assessment of the abdomen of the obstetrical client. Emphasis will be on the assessment of the physiological alterations occurring during the prenatal, the intrapartal, and the postpartal period. There will be a sequential focus upon:

1. The measurement of fundal height during pregnancy.
2. The palpation of fetal presentation and position during pregnancy and the intrapartal period.
3. The auscultation of fetal heart tones during pregnancy and the intrapartal period.
4. The palpation of uterine contractions during the intrapartal period.
5. The palpation of the involuting uterus.

The uterus, contained in the true pelvic cavity in its nonpregnant state, becomes a transient abdominal organ during the gestational period. Because abdominal palpation is one way of gathering data about the relationship between the fetal presentation and position and the maternal pelvis, fetopelvic relationships are included in this module. Additional and verifying data regarding fetopelvic relationships may be obtained by pelvic examination. Guidelines for the pelvic assessment of fetal presentation and position are included in Module 14.

You are to complete this module and pass the Posttest before the scheduled practicum for assessment of the obstetrical abdomen.

TERMINAL OBJECTIVES

Upon completion of this module you are expected to be able to:

1. State the purpose of fundal measurement throughout the prenatal period.
2. Given a diagram, label in centimeters from the symphysis pubis the approximate expected height of the gravid uterus at 12, 20, 28, 36, and 40 weeks gestation.
3. State three situations in which the fundal measurement might be inconsistent with the client's gestational period.
4. Define *fetal attitude, fetal lie, fetal presentation,* and *fetal position.*
5. State the most common form of fetal lie, presentation, and position.
6. State the significance of a transverse lie.
7. State the purpose of each of the four maneuvers of Leopold.
8. Given a diagram, identify each of the four maneuvers of Leopold.
9. Given a diagram of the maternal abdomen and pelvis and its fetus, identify the fetal presentation and position.
10. Palpate the pregnant abdomen for fetal presentation.
11. State the normal range of fetal heart tones.
12. State the gestational period in which fetal heart tones are audible with a fetoscope.
13. State the frequency in which fetal heart tones should be auscultated in early labor, in transition phase, and in the second stage of labor.
14. Demonstrate the use of a fetoscope.
15. Given a diagram, label the appropriate location for auscultation of fetal heart tones with
    a. The fetus in a vertex, left occiput anterior (LOA) position.
    b. The fetus in a frank breech presentation.
16. Differentiate between the uterine souffle, the fetal souffle, and the fetal heart tones.
17. Auscultate the pregnant abdomen for fetal heart tones and count the fetal heart beats for 1 minute.
18. Describe the method for determining the basal fetal heart rate.
19. State the cause and significance of early deceleration (type I dips), late deceleration (type II dips) and variable deceleration patterns of the fetal heartbeat.
20. Describe the technique for determining the frequency, duration, and strength of uterine contractions.
21. State the expected frequency, duration, and strength of uterine contractions in the first and second stages of labor.
22. Define *tetanic contraction* and state the significance of its occurrence to the maternal-fetal organism.
23. Evaluate correctly the uterine contractions of the intrapartal client.
24. Given a diagram of the maternal abdomen, label the expected approximate height of the fundus of the uterus immediately after delivery and on each of the 10 successive postpartum days.

25. State three conditions which explain variations in fundal height during the first 10 postpartal days.
26. Record accurately all data from the assessment of the obstetrical abdomen.

SUGGESTED ACTIVITIES

Read

Affonso, Dyanne D., and Ann Clark: "Application of Physiologic Perspectives, Ongoing Physical Evaluation (Growth of the Uterus)," *Childbearing: A Nursing Perspective,* Davis, Philadelphia, 1976.

AND

Jensen, Margaret Duncan, et al. *Maternity Care: The Nurse and The Family,* Mosby, St. Louis, 1977.

    "Maternal Physiology," changes in the genital tract (Uterus)
    "Normal Labor," (Fetal lie, presentation, and attitude); (Abdominal palpation and auscultation); (uterine contractions)
    "Third and Fourth Stages of Labor," separation and delivery of the placenta, Fourth Stage (Management)
    "The Puerperium," physiologic changes (genital tract: involution of the uterus)

OR

Dickason, Elizabeth J., and Martha Olsen Schult: *Maternal and Infant Care,* McGraw-Hill, New York, 1975.

    "Maternal Development," abdominal enlargement, "Process of Labor"
        Fetal positions
        Determination of fetal position
        Uterine contractions
        Fetal response to labor
        Third Stage of labor
        Fundus: Procedure for fundus check

OR

Ziegel, Erna, and Mecca Cranley: *Obstetric Nursing,* 7th ed., Macmillan, New York, 1978.

    "Maternal Physiologic Changes During Pregnancy," changes in the reproductive organs (uterine body), and estimating the probable date of delivery (growth of uterus)
    "Presentation and Position of the Fetus"
    "The Clinical Course and Mechanism of Labor and Delivery," clinical course of normal labor (characteristics of normal contractions)
    "Clinical Management During Labor," observations during labor (observation of the condition of the fetus), observations of the progress of labor (observation of uterine contractions)
    "Clinical Management of the Postpartum Family," postpartum physical assessment (abdomen-uterus)

View

Anatomy of the Female Pelvis and Reproductive Organs, Medical Electronic Educational Services filmstrip (MN-01).
Feto-Pelvic Relationships, Medical Electronic Educational Services filmstrip (MN-05).
Observing Contractions, Medical Electronic Educational Services filmstrip (LD-03).
Observing Fetal Heart Tones, Medical Electronic Educational Services filmstrip (LD-04).

Educational aid

Obstetrical Presentation and Position, Ross Clinical Education Aid No. 13.

Equipment

tape measure
fetoscope

VOCABULARY

acme	fetal presentation	Leopold's maneuvers
ballottement	fetal position	maternal souffle
contraction	fetal souffle	presenting part
decrement	flexion	station
early deceleration	funic souffle	symphysis pubis
engagement	fundus	tetanic contraction
extension	increment	type I dip
fetal attitude	involution	type II dip
fetal lie	late deceleration	variable deceleration

DECISION TABLE 10-1

If . . . → **Then . . .**

You need to review anatomy and physiology ⟹ Read the chapter concerning the reproductive system in your anatomy and physiology textbook.

The anatomy and physiology text is not complete enough ⟹ Oxorn, Harry, and William R. Foote: *Human Labor and Birth*, Appleton-Century-Crofts, New York, 1975.

⟹ MacDonald, Paul, and Jack Pritchard: *Williams Obstetrics*, Appleton-Century-Crofts, New York, 1976.

You need more information on variations in fundal height in pregnancy ⟹ Affonso, Dyanne D., and Ann Clark: *Childbearing: A Nursing Perspective*, Davis, Philadelphia, 1976.

You wish additional information on assessment of uterine contractions ⟹ Affonso, Dyanne D., and Ann Clark: *Childbearing: A Nursing Perspective*, Davis, Philadelphia, 1976.

⟹ McDonald, Paul, and Jack Pritchard: *Williams Obstetrics*, Appleton-Century-Crofts, New York, 1976.

⟹ Reeder, Sharon R., et al.: *Maternity Nursing*, Lippincott, Philadelphia, 1976.

You are having difficulty with fetopelvic relationships ⟹ *Obstetrical Presentation and Position*, Ross Clinical Education Aid (13).

⟹ Oxorn, Harry, and William R. Foote: *Human Labor and Birth*, Appleton-Century-Crofts, New York, 1975.

DECISION TABLE 10-1 (continued)

	⇒	MacDonald, Paul, and Jack Pritchard: *Williams Obstetrics*, Appleton-Century-Crofts, New York, 1976.
	⇒	Affonso, Dyanne D., and Ann Clark: *Childbearing: A Nursing Perspective*, Davis, Philadelphia, 1976.
You wish to do additional reading on monitoring of fetal heart rates	⇒	Hon, Edward H.: *An Introduction to Fetal Heart Rate Monitoring*, Harty Press, New Haven, 1969.
	⇒	"Intrapartum Evaluation of the Fetus" (supplement), *Journal of Obstetric, Gynecologic and Neonatal Nursing*, **5**(5), (September-October, 1976).
You would like to learn about fetal assessment in high-risk pregnancy	⇒	Tucker, Susan M.: *Fetal Monitoring*, Mosby, St. Louis, 1978.

POSTTEST

1. On Fig. 10-1, label the expected height of the fundus of the gravid uterus at 12, 20, 28, 36, and 40 weeks of gestation.

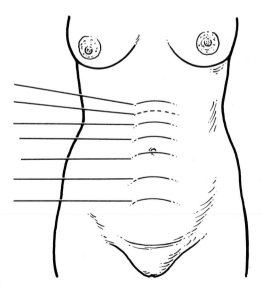

Figure 10-1

2. State *three* situations in which the fundal measurement might be inconsistent with the client's gestational period.

a. _____

b. _____

c. _____

3. Match the following terms and definitions:

_____ Lie

_____ Presentation

_____ Position

_____ Station

_____ Engagement

_____ Maneuvers of Leopold

_____ Fetal attitude

1. The part of the fetal body lying nearest to or having entered the true pelvis

2. A method of abdominal palpation for presentation and position of the fetus

3. The relationship of the parts of the fetal body to one another

4. The relation of an arbitrarily chosen point on the presenting part of the fetus to a specific quadrant of the maternal pelvis

5. The degree of fetal descent into the maternal pelvis

6. The relationship of the longitudinal axis of the fetus to the longitudinal axis of the mother

7. The passage of the presenting part of the fetus through the pelvic inlet

4. Using the diagrams in Fig. 10-2, indicate the *fetal attitude, lie, presentation,* and *position.*

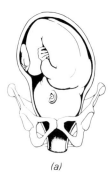
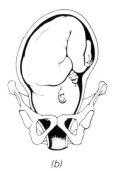

Figure 10-2

(a)   (b)

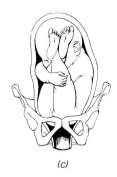
(c)

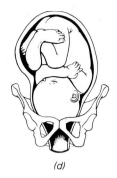
(d)

(*Source: Ross Clinical Education Aid No. 18,* Ross Laboratories, Columbus, Ohio.)

a. Attitude _____

   Lie _____

   Presentation _____

   Position _____

b. Attitude _____

   Lie _____

   Presentation _____

   Position _____

c. Attitude _____

   Lie _____

   Presentation _____

   Position _____

d. Attitude _____

   Lie _____

   Presentation _____

   Position _____

5. Using the photographs in Fig. 10-3 below, state which of the four maneuvers of Leopold is utilized and state briefly the purpose of each.

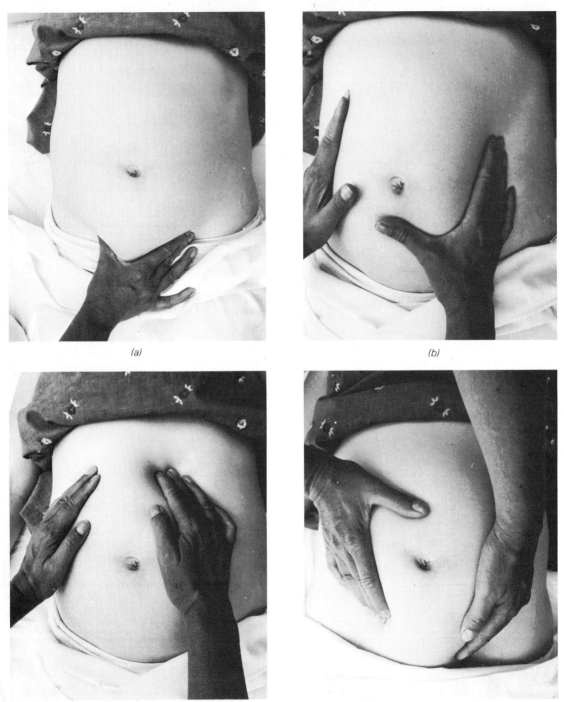

(a)

(b)

(c)   **Figure 10-3**   (d)

a. Maneuver _____

Purpose _____

_____

b. Maneuver _____

Purpose _____

_____

c. Maneuver _____

Purpose _____

_____

d. Maneuver _____

Purpose _____

_____

(*Source:* Photos from E. Dickason and M. Schult, *Maternal and Infant Care,* 2d ed., McGraw-Hill, New York, 1979.)

6. When performing Leopold's maneuvers on a client whose infant is in left occiput anterior (LOA) position, irregular fetal parts (arms and legs) are palpated on the mother's (*right, left*) side.

7. The normal range of fetal heart tones is _____.

8. On Fig. 10-4 , put an *X* at the point of maximum intensity of fetal heart tones of a fetus in the left occiput anterior (LOA) position.

9. On Fig. 10-5, put an *X* at the point of maximum intensity of fetal heart tones of a fetus in the right sacral anterior (RSA) position.

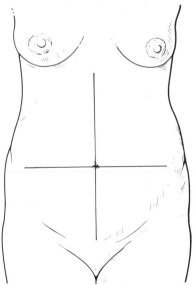

Figure 10-4

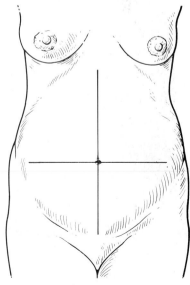

Figure 10-5

Write *true* or *false.* If *false,* correct by making statement true.

10. _____ The fetal heart tones can usually be heard with a fetoscope by 16 weeks of gestation.

11. _____ Uterine contractions are involuntary and are intermittent in nature.

12. _____ Uterine contractions during transition phase of first stage labor may normally last from 50 to 75 seconds.

13. _____ The intensity of a contraction is best measured by the client's subjective reports.

14. _____ A type II fetal heart dip begins during the increment of a contraction and is considered a normal deviation.

15. _____ The examiner can differentiate between the fetal heart beat and the uterine souffle by counting the mother's radial pulse.

16. _____ A transverse lie is an undeliverable vaginal presentation.

17. _____ The postpartal fundal check is done to determine the degree of uterine contraction and descent.

18. _____ The usual rate of postpartal fundal descent is 1 cm per day beginning the second day following delivery.

19. State *three* conditions which might account for variation in fundal height during the first 10 days postpartum.

a. _____

b. _____

c. _____

20. The nurse should palpate the fundus of the uterus at least every _____ minutes during the hour after delivery.

HEALTH HISTORY AND ASSESSMENT

This information should be obtained from the pregnant client in addition to a general health history which includes client identifying data, previous medical history, family medical history, and socioeconomic and cultural history (Module 1).

History of Obstetrical Client Pertinent to Assessment of the Abdomen

Remarks

1. First day of last menstrual period?
2. Pregnancy planned or unplanned?
3. If pregnancy unplanned, type of contraception at time of conception?
4. Previous menstrual period (first day of period before last menstrual period)?
5. Interval of usual menstrual cycle?
6. Number of previous pregnancies?
7. Number of miscarriages (abortions)?
8. Number of full-term births (9 months)?
9. Number of premature births (less than 8 ½ months)?
10. Number of living children?
11. Number of multiple births (twins, triplets)?
12. Complications of previous pregnancies (nausea and vomiting, bleeding, toxemia)?
13. Use of
    a. Tobacco (number of cigarettes per day)
    b. Alcohol (amount and kind of beverages consumed daily)
    c. Soft or hard drugs (LSD, marijuana, heroin)
    d. Prescription or nonprescription drugs
14. X-ray examination within past 6 months?
15. Illnesses and their treatment since last menstrual period?

16. Exposure to individuals with illnesses since last menstrual
period?
17. Method of previous deliveries
(vaginal or cesarean section)?
18. Length of previous labors?
19. Complications of previous labors
or deliveries?
20. Anesthetics with previous labors
or deliveries?
21. Weight of previously delivered infants?

Information about father of baby
1. Age?
2. Height?
3. Weight?
4. Blood type?
5. Any blood relationship of father
and mother? Yes _____ No _____
6. Chronic or acute health problems?

Additional information to be obtained if client in labor
1. Childbirth education?
2. Type of analgesia or anesthetic
planned?
3. Lightening (patient's subjective
report)?

   When occurred? _____

4. Show? Yes _____ No _____
5. Membranes:

   Intact? _____

   Ruptured? _____

   Date? _____ Time? _____
6. Onset of contractions?

7 . Time contractions became
regular?

8 . Last food intake (time, date, kind
of food)?

9 . Last time patient slept?

1 0 . Last voiding?

1 1 . Last defecation?

Additional information to be obtained if client has delivered

1 . Length of time since delivery?

2 . Complications of delivery?

3 . Method of placental delivery?*

Manual ____ Spontaneous ____

4 . Weight of infant?

5 . Oxytocic drugs received (dosage,
frequency)?*

6 . Fundal height, shape, and consistency immediately following
delivery?*

*Information may be obtained from client's medical record.

Physical Assessment of the Abdomen— Adaptations for the Obstetrical Client

Check (✔) if present, or fill in blanks as appropriate.

Prenatal and intrapartal assessment   Remarks

1 . Fundal height

_____ cms   _____ Normal

_____ Abnormal
(Corresponding weeks of ges-

tation) _____ Weeks of gestation

2 . Striae gravidarum _____

3 . Fetal movements

_____ Weeks of gestation (first
felt by mother)

_____ Weeks of gestation (felt by
other)

4. Presentation and position of fetus

_____ Weeks of gestation

Describe:

a. Location of fetal back (in relation to maternal abdomen)

b. Location of fetal small parts (in relation to maternal abdomen)

c. Location of fetal head (in relationship to maternal abdomen)

d. Location of fetal cephalic prominence (in relationship to maternal abdomen)

e. Presentation of fetus

f. Position of fetus

5. Auscultation of fetal heart tones

a. Presence of fetal heart sounds

Yes _____   No _____

Weeks of gestation _____

b. Rate of fetal heart sounds
_____ Beats per minute

c. Rhythm of fetal heart sounds

Regular _____ Irregular _____

d. Location of fetal heart sounds

_____

e. Presence of uterine souffle

Describe _____

f. Presence of fetal souffle

Describe _____

6. Uterine contractions (Periodic assessment of uterine contractions in labor is to be used together with assessment of cervical effacement and dilation and fetal descent for evaluation of overall progress of labor.) Record data from the palpation of uterine contractions for a 10-minute period:

Time contraction began	Duration of contraction	Intensity of contraction
_____	_____	_____
_____	_____	_____
_____	_____	_____
_____	_____	_____
_____	_____	_____
_____	_____	_____
_____	_____	_____
_____	_____	_____
_____	_____	_____

Summarize above data

Frequency   _____   _____

Intensity   _____   _____

Duration   _____   _____

Contractions becoming
longer in duration, intensity,
and more frequent
intervals?   Yes _____   No _____

Postpartal assessment   Remarks

1. Fundal height

   _____ cms

   _____ Hours/days after delivery

2. Fundal shape

   _____ Hours/days after delivery

3. Fundal consistency

   _____ Hours/days after delivery

4. Bladder distention

   Yes _____   No _____

Student_____

INSTRUCTOR'S GUIDE FOR EVALUATION OF STUDENT PERFOR-MANCE

Assessment of the Obstetrical Abdomen

Behaviors evaluated	Yes	No	Remarks
1. Assembles equipment needed			
2. Takes appropriate history for abdomen of the obstetrical client			
3. Explains procedure for examination to client			
4. Places client in supine position			
5. Drapes to expose abdomen only			
6. Inspects abdomen			
Measure of fundal height			
7. Measures distance from symphysis pubis to top of fundus			
Palpation for fetal presentation and position			
8. Performs maneuvers of Leopold in proper sequence:			
a. Palpates fundus with both hands			
b. Places both hands on sides of mother's abdomen			
c. Uses one hand to palpate presenting part above symphysis			
d. Faces client's feet, and pushes fingers down toward birth canal and palpates presenting part, feeling for cephalic prominence			
8. Determines fetal presentation and position before auscultating fetal heart tones			
Ausculation of fetal heart tones			
9. Warms fetoscope by rubbing with hands			
10. Uses fetoscope with proper placement of headpiece			
11. Auscultates for fetal heart tones in location of expected maximum intensity			
12. Counts rate of fetal heartbeat for 1 minute			
13. Places hand(s) over uterine fundus to palpate contractions			

Behaviors evaluated	Yes	No	Remarks
14. Leaves hand(s) quietly on fundus in order to detect intermittent uterine contraction and relaxation			
15. Notes the frequency, intensity, and duration of uterine contractions			
16. Assesses the frequency of contractions from the beginning of one until the beginning of the next one			
17. Assesses the duration of the contraction from its beginning to its end			
18. Assesses the strength of a uterine contraction upon the degree of indentation of the fundus at the peak of a contraction			
Palpation of postpartal uterus			
19. Measures fundal height in finger breadths from umbilicus on a postpartal client			
20. Supports lower segment of the uterus of a postpartal client before exerting any pressure on the fundus			
21. Records findings, using appropriate terminology			

Comments:

Instructor _____ Date _____

MODULE 11

ASSESSMENT OF THE MALE GENITALIA, HERNIAS, AND RECTUM

This instructional module is designed as a guide to assist you in learning a thorough and systematic approach to assessment of the male genitalia, hernias, and rectum. The health history includes the genitourinary and sexual history. Adaptations for assessing the pediatric and geriatric client are included. Through the use of some repetition, emphasis is upon assessment of age-related changes of the genitourinary system, although assessment techniques are similar to those for the adult.

The format for this module is similar to that of the previous modules. You are to complete the module and pass the Posttest before the scheduled laboratory period. The physical assessment may be performed on a model in the laboratory, if assessment of a male subject (infant, child, or adult) is not feasible. Important diagnostic findings can be missed if this part of the male physical examination is omitted.

If you have difficulty in completing the module contact your instructor.

PREREQUISITE OBJECTIVES

You should be able to:

1. Label the major organs and structures on a diagram of the male genitalia.
2. List the functions of the kidneys in maintaining homeostasis.
3. Describe the function of the testes, epididymis, vas deferens, seminal vesicles, and prostate gland.

TERMINAL OBJECTIVES

Upon completion of this module you are expected to be able to:

1. Define the vocabulary words accompanying this module.
2. Given an assessment form as a guide, take a health history pertinent to the genitourinary system of the male, using appropriate branching questions.
3. Discuss effective psychosocial approaches to interviewing the client to obtain a sexual history.
4. Given an assessment form as a guide, perform a systematic assessment of the male genitalia, rectum, and inguinal region.
5. Describe approaches which will aid in decreasing anxiety of the client and the nurse during the examination.
6. Using a model or a male subject, demonstrate inspection and palpation of the male genitalia, rectum, and inguinal region.
7. Describe the normal appearance and characteristics of the male penis and scrotum and the significance of abnormal findings.
8. Describe the procedure for palpation of femoral and inguinal hernias.
9. List significant observations to be made during inspection of the sacrococcygeal and perianal areas.
10. List significant findings to be noted during palpation of the anus, rectum, and prostate.
11. Describe the anatomical differences of the child that will be of significance to the examiner.
12. Describe techniques used in examination of the child.
13. Describe approaches to the child which will aid the nurse in preparing and positioning the child for examination.
14. Describe physiologic and functional changes in the male genitourinary system due to aging which should be considered in assessing the geriatric client.
15. Describe variations in physical findings among ethnic groups.
16. Record the data obtained from the health assessment, using correct medical terminology.

SUGGESTED ACTIVITIES

Read

Bates, Barbara: "Male Genitalia" and "Hernias, Anus, and Rectum," *A Guide to Physical Assessment,* Lippincott, Philadelphia, 1979.

OR

Malasanos, Lois, et al.: "Male Genitalia and Hernias," and "Rectosigmoid," *Health Assessment,* Mosby, St. Louis, 1977.

Alexander, Mary, and Marie Brown: "Male Genitalia," *Pediatric History Taking and Physical Diagnosis for Nurses,* McGraw-Hill, New York, 1979.

OR

Brown, Marie, and Mary Alexander: "Physical Examination: Male Genitalia," *Nursing '76,* 39–43 (February, 1976).

Caird, F. I., and T. G. Judge: "Genitourinary," *Assessment of the Elderly Patient,* Pitman, Calif., 1977.

OR

Saxon, Sue V., and Mary Jean Etten: "Urinary and Reproductive Systems" and "Sexuality," *Physical Change and Aging,* The Tiresias Press, New York, 1978.

View

Bates, Barbara: *Examination of Male Genitalia, Anus, and Rectum,* Lippincott, videotape, 9 min.

Educational Aids

Adam Teaching Model, OMNI Education (male genitalia and scrotum).
Prostate Palpation Simulator, Trainex Corporation.

Equipment

glove
lubricant
drape
penlight

PRETEST   With books closed, test your knowledge of anatomy of the male genitalia.

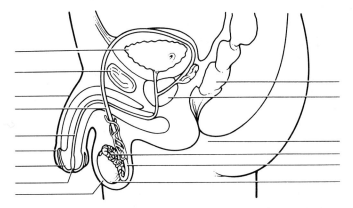

Figure 11-1

1. Label the structures on Fig. 11-1.
   a. Anus
   b. Rectum
   c. Bladder
   d. Epididymis
   e. Testis
   f. Scrotum
   g. Vas deferens
   h. Urethra
   i. Shaft of penis
   j. Glans
   k. Prepuce
   l. Urethral meatus
   m. Symphysis pubis
   n. Prostate

2. The rectum is approximately _____ to _____ inches long, and the anal canal is approximately _____ to _____ inches in length.

3. Name *four* functions of the kidneys in maintaining homeostasis.

    a. _____

    b. _____

    c. _____

    d. _____

Write *true* or *false.* If *false,* correct the statement to make it true.

4. _____ The epididymis plays a role in the maturation of sperm.

5. _____ The function of prostatic secretion is to aid in the motility of sperm.

6. _____ The central nervous system controls the dilatation of penile arteries and erection.

7. _____ The left testis is usually lower than the right.

8. _____ By birth, the testes have descended along the inguinal canal into the scrotum.

VOCABULARY   Descriptive terminology

cremasteric reflex	fistula	prepuce	spermatic cord
epididymis	impotent	prostate	strangulated
excoriation	incarcerated	pruritis	urethritis
fissure	polyp	smegma	vas deferens

Diagnostic terminology

benign prostatic hypertrophy (BPH)	epispadias	orchitis
chancre	gonorrhea	phimosis
chancroid	hematocele	pilonidal cyst
circumcision	hemorrhoid	priapism
condyloma acuminatum	herpes genitalis	syphilis
cryptorchism	hydrocele	varicocele
direct inguinal hernia	hypospadius	
epididymitis	indirect inguinal hernia	

DECISION TABLE 11-1

If . . .		Then . . .
You need additional pediatric references	⟹	Brown, Marie, and Mary Alexander: "Physical Examination: Part 14, Male Genitalia," *Nursing '76,* 39–43 (February, 1976).
	⟹	Scipien, Gladys M., et al.: *Comprehensive Pediatric Nursing,* 2d ed, McGraw-Hill, New York, 1979 (renal/GU history form included).
You need more information regarding sexuality	⟹	*Human Sexuality and Nursing Practice, No. 8, When the Topic is Sex,* Concept Media filmstrip.
	⟹	Burnside, Irene M.: *Nursing and the Aged,* McGraw-Hill, New York, 1976.
	⟹	Burnside, Irene M., Ed.: *Sexuality and Aging,* University of Southern California Press, Los Angeles, 1975.
You are not familiar with testicular self-examination	⟹	Murray, Barbara, and Linda J. Wilcox: "Testicular Self-Examination," *American Journal of Nursing,* 2074–2075 (December, 1978).

POSTTEST

1. List *three* abnormalities that can be detected on rectal examination in both male and female.

   a. _____

   b. _____

   c. _____

2. List *three* abnormalities of the prostate that can be detected by rectal examination.

   a. _____

   b. _____

   c. _____

3. To examine the prostate, the adult male should be in what position?

   _____

4. List *two* reasons why a rectal examination is especially important in the elderly male.

   a. _____

   b. _____

5. If the client complains of dysuria, the cause is frequently due to _____

_____ .

6. In elderly men, incontinence (or dribbling) accompanied by frequency and dif-

ficulty in starting micturition is usually due to _____ .

7. List *two* urinary symptoms that are major causes of disability in the elderly.

a. _____

b. _____

8. To examine for inguinal hernias, the male client should be in what position?

_____

9. In evaluating the newborn, evaluation of the rectal sphincter is important to de-

termine if _____ is

present. Suggest *one* method by which this evaluation may be accomplished.

_____

10. A _____ will present as a small bulge adjacent
and medial to the femoral artery about two fingerbreadths.

11. The cremasteric reflex of a child may cause apparent undescended testes. If the
testes are not felt in the scrotum, the child should climb onto the examining table
and assume what position?

_____

12. How would you phrase a question to determine the sexual drive, activity, and
satisfaction of a male client?

_____

13. List *two* health disorders that frequently interfere with sexual activity of the
geriatric client.

a. _____

b. _____

Write *true* or *false.* If *false,* correct the statement to make it true.

14. _____   The external inguinal ring is palpable through the abdominal wall.

15. _____   The foreskin should be retracted to examine the adult penis.

16. _____   The foreskin should not be retracted in examining the newborn.

17. _____   Pressure on the testes normally produces deep visceral pain.

18. _____   The prostate is palpated through the posterior rectal wall.

19. _____   The prostate is a sensitive organ.

20. _____   Urethral discharge is normal in the male.

21. _____   A femoral hernia is more common in males than females.

22. _____   An inguinal hernia is more common in males than females.

23. _____   Prostatic enlargement is a normal finding in older men.

HEALTH HISTORY AND ASSESSMENT

If the answer is yes, place a check (✓) at the left and provide further information in the Remarks column.

Adult Health History— Genitourinary Tract

Remarks

_____ Pain in kidney region?

_____ Get up at night to urinate?
   How many times?_____

_____ Swelling of hands or feet?
   In the evening? _____
   In the morning?_____

_____ Blood or pus in urine?

_____ Albumin in urine?

_____ Sugar in urine?

_____ Frequent urination?

_____ Burning or pain on urination?

_____ Pain over bladder?

_____ Trouble starting urine?

_____ Urinary stream weak?

_____ Hard to empty bladder completely?

_____ Hard to control urine when coughing or sneezing?

_____ History of stones?

_____ Any discharge, irritation, or lesion?

_____ Any scrotal pain or swelling?

_____ Any hernias?

_____ Any infection or surgery of prostate?

Sexual history

_____ Age of onset of sexual activity? _____

_____ Presently sexually active?

_____ Sexually active with more than one partner?

_____ Homosexual experiences?

_____ Any concerns about present level of sexual functioning?

_____ Difficulty with maintaining erection or premature ejaculation?

_____ Methods of birth control used?

_____ History of venereal disease?

Pediatric Adaptations— History

_____ No bladder control?
       Age of bladder control?_____

_____ Wets bed at night?

_____ Frequent sore throats?

_____ Swelling around eyes?

_____ Itching or scratching around rectum?

Geriatric Adaptations— History

_____ Dribbling or inability to control urine?

    _____ Any warning of the need to urinate?

    _____ Toilet facilities easily accessible?

    _____ Accompanied by another illness?

    _____ Accompanied by constipation?

_____ Frequent urination?

    _____ Small amounts of urine?

    _____ Large amounts of urine?

    _____ At night?

_____ Drink coffee, tea, or other fluids late in the evening?

_____ Reduced urine volume?

_____ Taking any diuretics?
       Name, dosage, and time of day taken?_____

_____ Any treatment or surgery for prostatic enlargement or cancer?

_____ Surgery for hernia repair?

_____ Wear a truss?

_____ History of hemorrhoids?

_____ Decline in frequency or satisfaction of sexual activity?

_____ Health disorder that interferes
with sexual function?

_____ Impotence?

_____ Difficulty retracting foreskin?

Adult Physical Assessment— Male Genitalia, Rectum, and Anus

Check (✓) if normal, _NE_ if not examined, _X_ if abnormal. Describe abnormal findings.

Genitalia   Description

_____ Penis: Circumcised

_____ No discharge, inflammation,
or swelling

_____ No ulcers, scars, or nodules

_____ Urethral meatus in correct
location

_____ Scrotum: No masses, ulceration, or lesions

_____ No inflammation or edema of
scrotum

_____ Testes and epididymis: Normal
size and consistency

_____ No inguinal or femoral hernia

_____ Prostate: Soft, nontender, no
enlargement or nodules

Rectum and anus

_____ No inflammation, rash, or
excoriation

_____ No lesions, fissures, or hemorrhoids

_____ No masses

_____ Sphincter tone good

_____ No bleeding

_____ No pilonidal cyst

_____ Stool _____

_____ No occult blood

Pediatric Adaptations— Physical

_____ Cremasteric reflex present

_____ No hypospadias, epispadias, phimosis

_____ Testes descended

_____ Urinary stream unrestricted

_____ Prostate no larger than 1 cm (if indicated)

_____ Circumcision healed

_____ Patent anal opening

_____ No abnormality of color of anus (no dark ring)

_____ Pubic hair: Pattern _____

_____ Genital development appropriate for age

_____ Testes of equal size

Geriatric Adaptations— Physical

_____ No fecal impaction

_____ No phimosis

_____ No scrotal edema

_____ Prostate edges palpable

_____ No nodules of prostate

Treatment, disposition, and recommendations regarding abnormal findings:

Student_____

INSTRUCTOR'S GUIDE FOR EVALUATION OF STUDENT PERFOR-MANCE

Assessment of the male genitalia, hernias, and rectum

Behaviors evaluated	Yes	No	Remarks
1. Assembles equipment needed			
2. Takes appropriate genitourinary and sexual history*			
3. Asks branching questions as appropriate			
4. Explains procedure for examination to client			
5. Places client in standing position, if adult			
6. Drapes to allow minimal exposure of client			
7. Places glove on examining hand			
8. Inspects penis			
9. Palpates penis			
10. Inspects scrotum			
11. Palpates scrotum			
12. Palpates inguinal areas			
13. Palpates inguinal rings, instructing client to cough or bear down			
14. Palpates femoral areas			
15. Asks client to lean over examining table			
16. Inspects anal and perianal region			
17. Lubricates gloved fingers			
18. Palpates rectum in a circular motion			
19. With palm down, gently palpates prostate			
20. As finger is withdrawn, inspects for blood, discharge, or fecal material			
21. Tests for occult blood			
22. Cleanses anal region			
23. Records findings, using appropriate terminology			

*Evaluated on previously submitted history.

Instructor _____ Date _____

MODULE 12

ASSESSMENT OF THE BREASTS AND AXILLAE

This instructional module is designed as a guide to assist you in learning a systematic approach for the assessment of the breasts and axillae. Emphasis is on taking an appropriate health history and learning inspection and palpation of the breasts and axillae. Adaptations for the assessment of the obstetrical client are included in Part 2 of this module.

    The format for this unit is similar to previous modules. You are to complete this module and pass the Posttest before the scheduled laboratory period or clinical practicum for assessment of the breasts and axillae.

PREREQUISITE OBJECTIVES

You should be able to:

1. State the anatomical location of the female breasts in relationship to the rib cage.
2. Given a diagram, identify the following external features of the female breast:
    a. Areolar (sebaceous) gland
    b. Nipple
    c. Areola
    d. Breast
3. Given a diagram, identify the following components of breast tissue:
    a. Glandular tissue
    b. Fibrous tissue
    c. Fat
4. State the function of the ducts of the breast.

5. Name the three groups of lymph nodes which drain into the central axillary nodes.

TERMINAL OBJECTIVES

Upon completion of this module you are expected to be able to:

1. Define the terms on the accompanying vocabulary list.
2. State the pertinent observations to be made regarding the size and symmetry, the contour, and the skin characteristics of the breast.
3. State the significance of the following findings which can be gained from inspection of the nipples of the female breast:
   a. Size and shape
   b. Inversion
   c. Presence of rashes
   d. Presence of discharge
   e. Direction in which nipples are pointed
4. Describe normal findings expected from palpation of the breasts.
5. Explain the underlying rationale for the presence of engorgement of breast tissue in a newborn infant.
6. List six characteristics to be described about nodules palpated during breast examination.
7. Given an assessment guide, take a health history pertinent to the breasts and axillae.
8. Describe the appropriate technique for examination of female breasts and axillae.
9. Demonstrate an assessment of the female breasts and axillae by utilizing appropriate inspection and palpation techniques.
10. Record data, using appropriate terminology to describe findings.
11. Describe the changes in breast tissue related to the aging process.

SUGGESTED ACTIVITIES

Read

Bates, Barbara: "Breasts and Axillae," "Pediatric Physical Examination," and "The Thorax," *A Guide to Physical Assessment,* Lippincott, Philadelphia, 1979.
OR
Malasanos, Lois, et al.: "Assessment of the Breasts," *Health Assessment,* Mosby, St. Louis, 1977.

View

Bates, Barbara: *Physical Assessment Examinations—Breast,* Lippincott videotape, 7 min.

Equipment

model of breast
cape or gown

PRETEST   With books closed, test your knowledge of the anatomy of the female breast and axillae.

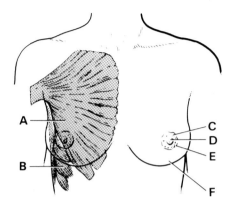

Figure 12-1

1. Label the structures shown in Figure 12-1.

    a. _____

    b. _____

    c. _____

    d. _____

    e. _____

    f. _____

2. Label the following structures on Fig. 12-2:

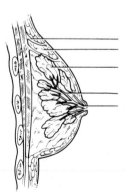

Figure 12-2

    a. Fat
    b. Glandular tissue
    c. Duct
    d. Opening of duct on nipple
    e. Suspensory ligament

3. Label the following structures on Fig. 12-3:

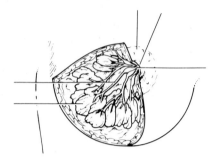

Figure 12-3

   a. Opening of duct on nipple

   b. Areola

   c. Duct

   d. Glandular tissue

   e. Nipple

4. The female breast lies between the _____

   and _____ ribs.

VOCABULARY

Descriptive terminology

acini	Montgomery's tubercles	peau d'orange
areola	nipple deviation	retraction
axillary tail tissue	nipple inversion	supernumerary tissue

Diagnostic terminology

adenofibroma	fibrocystic disease	Paget's disease
adenocarcinoma	lymphadenitis	
cystic disease	mastitis	

POSTTEST

1. The female breast lies between the _____ and

   _____ ribs.

2. Breast tissue has *three* principal components. Name and describe the location of each.

   a. _____

   b. _____

   c. _____

3. Inspection of the female breast and nipples includes observation of the

   a. 1, 2, 4
   b. 1, 2, 3
   c. 3, 4, 5
   d. All of these

   1. Size and symmetry
   2. Contour
   3. Appearance of the skin
   4. Discharge
   5. Ulcerations

4. Explain *two* methods of localizing and describing findings of breast examination.

   a. _____

   b. _____

5. The purpose of placing a pillow under the client's shoulder on the side of the breast being examined is to _____

   _____ .

6. List *six* characteristics to be described about nodules palpated during breast examination:

   a. _____

   b. _____

   c. _____

   d. _____

   e. _____

   f. _____

7. The purpose of asking the client to raise her arms over her head, and to press her hands against her hips during examination of the breast is to _____

   _____ .

8. Dimpling of the breast skin is suggestive of _____

   _____ .

9. Edema of the skin over the breast, produced by lymphatic blockage, is manifested by a thickened skin with enlarged pores and is referred to as _____

   _____ .

10. Erosion or ulceration of the nipple and areola is suggestive of _____

    _____ .

Write *true* or *false.* If *false,* correct the statement to make it true.

11. _____ Inversion of the nipple is a normal variant.

12. _____ Dermatitis of the nipple and areola is a common, normal occurrence.

13. _____ Deviation (pointing) of the nipple is suggestive of cancer.

14. _____ Nipple flattening or retraction is associated with breast cancer.

15. _____ Nipple discharge may be associated with cancer.

16. _____ Malignant breast nodules are usually tender to touch.

17. _____ Malignant breast nodules are frequently very mobile.

18. _____ Malignant breast nodules are clearly delineated from surrounding tissues.

19. _____ The breasts of the female infant are normally edematous for a few days following delivery.

20. _____ Inspection of the axillae is made to identify the presence of rashes or infection.

21. _____ Palpation of the axillae is best achieved with the client in a sitting position.

22. _____ Enlarged axillary nodes are suggestive of axillary metastases of breast cancer or lymphadenitis.

23. _____ Breast development precedes menarche.

24. Name the four sets of lymph nodes to be palpated in the axillae:

a. _____

b. _____

c. _____

d. _____

HEALTH HISTORY AND ASSESSMENT

If the answer is yes, place a check (✔) at the left and provide further information in the Remarks column.

Breasts and Axillae — History

Remarks

_____ Enlargement, tenderness, or lumps?

_____ Nipple discharge?

_____ Monthly breast examination?

_____ Any lumps or tenderness in axillae?

_____ Any skin irritation?

Physical Assessment

Check (✔) if normal, *NE* if not examined, *X* if abnormal. Describe abnormal findings.

Description

_____ Size

_____ Symmetrical

_____ No supernumerary nipple

_____ Smooth contour, no dimpling or flattening

_____ No masses or tenderness

_____ Nipples erect, no discharge

_____ Lymph nodes nontender, non-palpable

_____ Lateral

_____ Subscapular (posterior)

_____ Pectoral (anterior)

_____ Central

Geriatric Adaptation — Physical

_____ Breast tissue loose, atrophied

Male Adaptation — Physical

_____ No gynecomastia

Pediatric Adaptation— Physical

_____ Breast engorgement (newborn)

_____ No breast development

_____ Breast development appropriate to age

_____ No axillary hair

_____ Presence of axillary hair

Disposition, recommendations, or treatment of abnormal findings:

Student_____

INSTRUCTOR'S GUIDE FOR EVALUATION OF STUDENT PERFOR-MANCE

Assessment of the Breasts and Axillae, Part 1

Behaviors evaluated	Yes	No	Remarks
1. Assembles equipment needed			
2. Asks client to disrobe to the waist			
3. Places client in sitting position			
4. Inspects breasts for			
a. Size and symmetry			
b. Contour			
c. Appearance of skin			
d. Direction in which nipples point			
e. Rashes			
f. Ulcerations			
g. Discharge			
5. Reinspects contour of breast for contour or dimpling, asking client to			
a. Put arms over head			
b. Then press hands against hips			
c. Lean forward (with support) if breasts are pendulous			
6. Places client in supine position with a small pillow under shoulder on side being examined			
7. Palpates breast systematically with pads of fingers and compresses breast tissue gently against chest wall			
8. Notes normal variations of breast tissue:			
a. Premenstrual fullness			
b. Elasticity of young person's breast			
9. Describes characteristics of nodules present:			
a. Size			
b. Location			
c. Shape			
d. Consistency			
e. Mobility			
f. Tenderness			
10. Assesses the axillae with client in sitting position			

Behaviors evaluated	Yes	No	Remarks
11. Inspects axillae for rash or infection			
12. Palpates axillae with fingers beginning from apex of axillae and continuing over rib cage and humerus			
13. Records all data accurately using appropriate terminology			

Instructor _____   Date _____

Part 2 of this instructional module is designed as a guide to assist you in learning a thorough and systematic approach for obtaining a health history and making an assessment of the breasts of the obstetrical client. Emphasis will be on the physiological alterations occurring during the prenatal and postnatal periods.

The format of Part 2 of this module is similar to that of previous modules. You are to complete this module and pass the Posttest before the scheduled practicum for assessment of the obstetrical client. If you have any questions, contact your instructor.

TERMINAL OBJECTIVES

Upon completion of this module you are expected to be able to:

1. Describe the changes which take place in the breasts during pregnancy.
2. State which observations of the breasts are important for the nurse to make during pregnancy.
3. State the purpose of the nurse's assessing the postpartal client's breasts.
4. Describe the changes which take place postpartally in the breasts of a woman who is not breast-feeding her infant.
5. Describe the changes which take place postpartally in the breast of a woman who is breast-feeding her infant.
6. Define *colostrum.*
7. Describe inversion of the nipple and state its significance to the obstetrical client.
8. Describe the anatomy and physiology of lactation.
9. State the significance to the postpartal client of engorgement of the breasts.
10. Describe the appearance of fissured nipples.
11. Using an assessment form as a guide, correctly assess the breasts of the prenatal and postpartal client.
12. Define *mastitis.*
13. State the relationship of mastitis to breast-feeding.

SUGGESTED ACTIVITIES

Read

Ziegel, Erna, and Mecca Cranley: "Breast Changes in Pregnancy" and "Breast Changes During the Puerperium," *Obstetric Nursing,* Macmillan, New York, 1978.

OR

Benson, Margaret Duncan, et al.: "Maternal Physiology—Breast Changes," "The Puerperium, Patient Care Objectives—Breast," and "Infant Nutrition, Lactation," *Maternity Care: The Nurse and the Family,* Mosby, St. Louis, 1977.

OR

Dickason, Elizabeth J., and Martha Olsen Schult: "The Process of Recovery," "Breast Care," "Infant Feeding," "Breast Changes During Pregnancy," and "Mechanism of Lactation," *Maternal and Infant Care,* McGraw-Hill, New York, 1975.

VOCABULARY

Descriptive terminology

colostrum	fissures	lactating
engorgement	inversion of the nipple	letdown reflex

Diagnostic terminology

mastitis

POSTTEST

1. Name *five* changes which occur in the breasts during pregnancy.

   a.

   b.

   c.

   d.

   e.

2. Colostrum may be expressed from the nipples of a pregnant woman as early as

   the _____ month of gestation.

3. Colostrum is secreted from the breasts of women for the first _____ days after delivery.

4. Select the *two* terms which are most descriptive of colostrum.

   a. Thin   b. Clear   c. Yellowish   d. White   e. Thick

5. Define *breast engorgement*.

6. Breast engorgement usually disappears in _____ to _____ hours after milk begins to come into the breasts.

7. Describe the appearance of the breasts during the engorgement period.

8. The breasts may feel_____ and_____ to the examiner during the engorgement period.

9. Explain the significance of an inverted nipple to the nursing mother.

10. Define *mastitis*.

11. Name *three* symptoms of mastitis.

    a.

    b.

    c.

12. Explain the significance of mastitis to the breast-feeding mother.

HEALTH HISTORY AND ASSESSMENT

Adult Health History: Female Breasts and Axillae — Adaptations for the Obstetrical Client

If the answer is yes, place a check (✓) at the left and provide further information in the Remarks column.

Information to be obtained if pregnant   Remarks

_____ Months of gestation? _____

_____ Use of brassiere?

      Note adequate support

      Comfortable? Yes___ No___

      Throbbing? Yes____ No____

      Tingling? Yes_____ No_____

_____ Color changes of areola (noted by client)?

_____ Discharge from nipples (noted by client)? Yes_____ No_____

      Describe _____

_____ Plans for infant feeding?

_____

Information to be obtained postpartally

Puerperal day? _____ 1

                 _____ 2

                 _____ 3

                 _____ 4

                 _____ 5

                 _____ Other

_____ Antilactogenic agents received if not breast-feeding? Date received? (Information may be collected from medical record.)

_____ Fluid intake?

_____ Breast support? Describe.

_____

_____ Colostrum present?

      Yes_____ No_____

_____ Milk present? Yes____ No____

_____ Tenderness or pain? Yes_____

      No_____ Describe_____

_____

_____ Engorgement (as reported by client)?

a. Redness? Yes_____ No_____

b. Firmness? Describe_____

c. Cracks in nipples?
   Yes_____ No_____

Physical Assessment of the Breasts and Axillae— Adaptations for the Obstetrical Client

Check (✔) if normal, *NE* if not examined, *X* if abnormal. Describe all abnormal findings.

Description

_____ Size _____

_____ Breast-feeding

_____ Colostrum

_____ Milk

_____ Engorgement

_____Pain

_____Tenderness

_____Cracks in nipples

_____Color

_____ Inversion of nipples

_____ Lymph nodes nontender, non-palpable

Student_____

INSTRUCTOR'S GUIDE FOR EVALUATION OF STUDENT PERFOR-MANCE

Assessment of the Female Breasts and Axillae, Part 2

Behaviors evaluated	Yes	No	Remarks
1. Assembles equipment needed			
2. Washes hands before assessing breasts			
3. Assesses the breasts of the pregnant client for			
a. Increase in size			
b. Firmness			
c. Prominence of nipples			
d. Color of areola			
e. Appearance of veins			
f. Size of Montgomery's glands			
4. Assesses the breasts of the postpartal client for			
a. Size			
b. Presence of colostrum			
c. Milk			
d. Engorgement			
e. Tenderness			
f. Cracks in nipples			
g. Color			
h. Inversion of nipples			
5. Assesses lymph nodes for enlargement			

Instructor _____ Date _____

MODULE 13

ASSESSMENT OF THE FEMALE GENITALIA, PART 1

This instructional module is designed as a guide to assist you in learning a systematic approach for the assessment of the female external and internal genitalia. Emphasis is on taking an appropriate health history and learning inspection of the female genitalia. Objectives for the advanced student include: (1) inspection of the vagina and cervix, (2) the performance of a bimanual examination, and (3) obtaining a Papanicolaou. Adaptations for the assessment of the obstetrical client are included in Module 14.

The format for this unit is similar to that of previous modules. You are to complete this module and pass the Posttest before the scheduled laboratory period or clinical practicum for assessment of the genitalia.

PREREQUISITE OBJECTIVES

You should be able to:

1. Describe the events of the normal menstrual cycle.
2. Label the anatomical structures of the external and internal female genitalia on a diagram.

TERMINAL OBJECTIVES

Upon completion of this module you are expected to be able to:

1. Define the terms in the Vocabulary for this module.
2. Given an assessment form as a guide, take a health history pertinent to the female genitalia.

257

3. Discuss effective approaches to interviewing the client to obtain a sexual history.

4. Describe the anatomical differences of the child which should be considered when making an assessment of the female genitalia.

5. Describe anatomical and functional changes in the female reproductive system due to aging which should be considered when assessing the geriatric client.

6. List the observations which should be made upon inspection of the external genitalia.

7. Discuss the preparation of the patient for examination of the genitalia.

8. Describe the technique for assessment of the Bartholin's glands.

9. Describe the technique for assessment of the support of the vaginal outlet.

10. Describe the technique for inserting a vaginal speculum.

11. State the observations to be made while inspecting the cervix.

12. State the source of three specimens which are collected for the Papanicolaou smear.

13. Describe the procedure for obtaining a Papanicolaou smear.

14. State the observations to be made while inspecting the vagina.

15. State the purpose of a bimanual pelvic examination.

16. Describe the procedure for performing a bimanual pelvic examination.

17. State the expected findings of a bimanual pelvic examination.

18. Given an assessment form as a guide, perform an assessment of the female external and internal genitalia.

19. Record all assesssment findings, using appropriate terminology.

SUGGESTED ACTIVITIES

Read

Bates, Barbara: "Female Genitalia," "Pediatric Physical Examination," and "Genitalia of Infant," *A Guide to Physical Assessment,* Lippincott, Philadelphia, 1979.

OR

Malasanos, Lois, et al.: "Assessment of the Female Genitalia," *Health Assessment,* Mosby, St. Louis, 1977.

Alexander, Mary, and Marie Brown: "Female Genitalia," *Pediatric History Taking and Physical Diagnosis for Nurses,"* McGraw-Hill, New York, 1979.

Saxon, Sue V., and Mary Jean Etten: "The Reproductive System," *Physical Change and Aging,* The Tiresias Press, New York, 1978.

View

Bates, Barbara: *Physical Assessment Examinations—Female Genitalia,* Lippincott, videotape, 10 min.

Educational aid

Gynny Pelvic Teaching Model, Omni Education.

Equipment

gloves
speculum
water for lubricant
water-soluble lubricant
light
Pap materials
    slides
    fixative
     Pap sticks
     cotton applicator

PRETEST

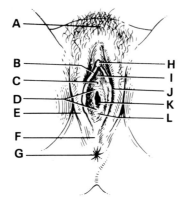

Figure 13-1

1. Label the structures shown in Fig. 13-1.

a. _____

b. _____

c. _____

d. _____

e. _____

f. _____

g. _____

h. _____

i. _____

j. _____

k. _____

l. _____

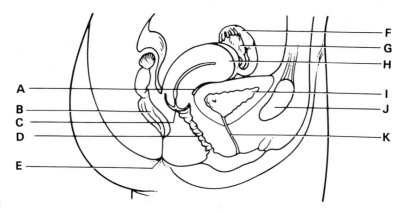

Figure 13-2

2. Label the structures in Fig. 13-2.

a. _____

b. _____

c. _____

d. _____

e. _____

f. _____

g. _____

h. _____

i. _____

j. _____

k. _____

3. Name the sequential events of the normal menstrual cycle.

VOCABULARY   **Descriptive terminology**

Bartholin's glands	introitus	retroflexion of uterus
cervix	isthmus of uterus	retroversion of uterus
climacteric	mons veneris	Skene's glands
clitoris	Nabothian (retention) cysts	uterus
endocervical	ovary	vagina
erosion	perineum	vaginitis
eversion	prepuce	vestibule
fallopian tube	prolapse	vulvitis
fornix	pudendum	
hymen	rectouterine pouch	

Diagnostic terminology

chancre

condolymata accuminatum

cystocele

gonorrhea

hemophilus vaginitis

herpes genitalis

Monilia (*Candida*)

myoma

ovarian cyst

pediculosis pubis

pelvic inflammatory disease

polyp

rectocele

senile vaginitis

syphilis

Trichomonas vaginitis

DECISION TABLE 13-1

If . . .		Then . . .
You prefer a programmed-learning approach	⟹	"Physical Assessment: Examination of the Female Pelvis: Part I," *American Journal of Nursing*, 1717-1726 (October, 1978).
For a thorough discussion of the female genitalia and pelvic examination	⟹	Prior, John A., and Jack S. Silberstein: "Genitalia," *Physical Diagnosis*, Mosby, St. Louis, 1977.
You are interested in learning about menstrual disorders	⟹	DeGowin, Richard L.: *Diagnostic Examination*, Macmillan, New York, 1969.
You need more information related to human sexuality	⟹	Adams, Georgia: "The Sexual History as an Integral Part of the Patient History," *MCN, The American Journal of Maternal Child Nursing*, 1(3): 170-175 (May-June, 1976).
	⟹	Zalar, Marianne K.: Sexual Counseling for Pregnant Couples, *MCN, The American Journal of Maternal Child Nursing*, 1(3):176-181 (May-June, 1976).
You want to know more about sexuality in the elderly	⟹	Burnside, Irene Mortenson, Ed.: *Sexuality and Old Age*, McGraw-Hi New York, 1976.
	⟹	Yeaworth, Rosalee C., and Joyce S Friedeman: "Sexuality in Later Life, *Nursing Clinics of North America*, 565-573 (September, 1975).
You wish to learn how to help your client during her first pelvic exam	⟹	Wells, Gail M.: "Reducing the Threat of a First Pelvic Exam," *MCN, The American Journal of Maternal Child Nursing*, 2(5):304-306 (September-October, 1977).

DECISION TABLE 13-1 (continued)

If . . .		Then . . .
You need information on venereal herpes	⟹	Edwards, Martha Shatley: "Venereal Herpes: A Nursing Overview," *JOGN Nursing,* **7**(5):7-18 (September–October, 1978).
You need more information on recognizing symptoms of gonorrhea or syphilis	⟹	Romney, Seymour L., et al.: "Specific Problems," *Gynecology and Obstetrics, The Health Care of Women,* McGraw-Hill, New York, 1975.
You need more information on recognizing symptoms of condylomas	⟹	Romney, Seymour L., et al.: "Specific Problems," *Gynecology and Obstetrics, The Health Care of Women,* McGraw-Hill, New York, 1975.
You need more information on recognizing symptoms of vaginitis (monilia, trichimonas)	⟹	Romney, Seymour L., et al.: "Specific Problems," *Gynecology and Obstetrics, The Health Care of Women,* McGraw-Hill, New York, 1975.

POSTTEST

1. There is frequently a bloody mucoid vaginal discharge during a female infant's first week of life due to _____

_____ .

Write *true* or *false.* If *false,* correct the statement to make it true.

2. _____ The genitalia of the female infant are normally edematous for a few days following delivery.

3. _____ Fusion of the labia minora is common in female infants.

4. _____ The internal pelvic exam is a routine part of the assessment of the genitalia of the preadolescent.

5. The primary purpose of examination of the genitalia of the newborn is to

_____ .

6. The position which permits the best visualization of the female external genitalia is the _____ position.

7. List *four* findings to be observed on the inspection of the female external genitalia.

   a. _____

   b. _____

   c. _____

   d. _____

8. Describe the technique for examining the Bartholin's glands.

_____

_____

9. Assessment of cystoceles is facilitated by asking the client to:
   a. Strain down
   b. Squeeze buttocks together

10. An acceptable lubricant for use in pelvic examination accompanied by cytological studies is _____ .

11. Insertion of the vaginal speculum is easiest with the blades held in a _____ position.

12. After insertion of the speculum into the vagina, the blades of the speculum should be rotated into a _____ position.

13. List *five* observations to make while inspecting the cervix.

    a. _____

    b. _____

    c. _____

    d. _____

    e. _____

14. When the cervix is located anteriorly, the uterus is probably in a _____ _____ position.

15. Specimens for cervical cytology may be taken from *three* locations. Name them.

    a. _____

    b. _____

    c. _____

16. When the cervix has been removed, cytology specimens are taken from the _____ and the _____ .

17. List *three* findings to be noted while inspecting the vagina.

    a. _____

    b. _____

    c. _____

18. Palpation of the uterus by bimanual examination reveals
    a. 1, 2, 5   1. Size
    b. 2, 3, 5   2. Shape
    c. 1, 3, 4   3. Consistency
    d. All of these   4. Mobility
                        5. Tenderness

19. Why is it recommended that gloves be changed between vaginal and rectal examinations? _____

_____

Write *true* or *false*. If *false*, correct the statement to make it true.

20. _____ Many vaginal orifices will readily admit a single examining finger.

21. _____ If a virginal vaginal orifice will not admit a single finger, a bimanual examination can be performed with one finger in the rectum.

22. In the space provided below, draw a
    a. Parous cervix
    b. Nulliparous cervix
    c. Lacerated cervix
    d. Polyp
    e. Erosion

23. Early carcinomas of the cervix are clinically indistinguishable from _____

_____ .

The following pathology-related questions are for the advanced student.

24. Trichimonas vaginitis is characterized by a profuse discharge, _____

in color, and _____ in consistency.

25. The discharge of monilia vaginitis is characteristically _____ .

26. Vaginal mucosa of a patient with candidas is _____

_____ .

27. Definitive diagnosis of vaginitis is dependent upon _____ .

28. The vaginal mucosa of an elderly woman may be _____

and _____ .

29. In varying degrees of uterine prolapse, the cervix is located in which of the following locations:

_____ first degree   a. Cervix and vagina protrude through introitus
_____ second degree   b. Within vagina
_____ third degree   c. Cervix at the introitus

30. Myomas of the uterus present clinically (upon examination) as _____

_____ or _____ .

Write *true* or *false.* If *false,* correct the statement to make it true.

31. _____ In moderate degrees of uterine retroversion, the fundus may not be accessible to either examining hand.

32. _____ In marked uterine retroversion the fundus may be felt through the rectum.

33. _____ Retroflexion of the uterus, a backward angulation of the body of the uterus in relationship to the cervix, is a variation of the normal uterine position.

34. _____ Ovarian tumors are smooth and compressible to the examiner's fingers.

35. _____ Cysts on the ovary feel solid and nodular to the examiner's fingers.

36. Movement of the cervix (by the examiner) produces pain in the patient with

_____ or _____ .

HEALTH HISTORY AND ASSESSMENT

If the answer is yes, place a check ($\checkmark$) at the left and provide further information in the Remarks column.

Adult Health History: Female External and Internal Genitalia

Genitourinary

Remarks

_____ Pain in kidney region?

_____ Get up at night to urinate? How many times?

_____ Swelling of hands or feet?
    In the morning? _____
    In the evening? _____

_____ Blood or pus in urine?

_____ Albumin in urine?

_____ Sugar in urine?

_____ Frequent urination?

_____ Burning or pain on urination?

_____ Pain over bladder?

_____ Trouble starting urine?

_____ Hard to empty bladder completely?

_____ Hard to control urine when coughing or sneezing?

_____ History of stones?

_____ Sexually active?

_____ Method of contraception?

_____ Painful intercourse?

_____ Experiencing orgasm?

_____ History of venereal disease?

_____ Common vaginal infections?

_____ Menses:

    Date of last period? _____

    Age began? _____

    Now occurs about every
    _____ days

    Number of days of flow? ____

    _____Flooding? Number of
        pads per day?_____

    _____Irregular?

    _____Painful? If so, how
        relieved? _____

_____ Spotting between periods?

_____ Age when "change of life" started? _____

_____ Hot flashes?

_____ Any history of trouble with female organs?

_____ Use of hormones? If yes,

       What? _____

       How long? _____

_____ Did mother take DES during pregnancy?

_____ Pregnancies? Number _____

_____ Complications of pregnancy?

_____ Any miscarriages?

_____ Vaginal itching?

_____ Increase in amount of vaginal discharge?

_____ Taken antibiotics in past month?

_____ Taking birth control pills?

_____ Date of last Pap smear? _____

       _____ Results

Geriatric Adaptations— History

_____ Decline in frequency or satisfaction of sexual activity?

_____ Health disorder that interferes with sexual function?

_____ Any vaginal bleeding or discharge since menopause?

_____ Inability to control urine?

       _____ Any warning of the desire to urinate?

       _____ Accompanied by another illness?

_____ Toilet facilities easily accessible?

_____ Reduced urine volume?

_____ Taking any diuretics? Name, dosage, time of day taken?

**Pediatric
Adaptations—
History
Infant/Child**

_____ Bladder Control
    Age _____
_____ Bedwetting at night

**Preadolescent/
Adolescent**

_____ Instructed on menstruation?
_____ Menses begun?
    Age began _____
_____ Sexually active?
    Age began _____
_____ Instructed on contraceptives?

**Adult Physical
Assessment—
Female
External and
Internal
Genitalia**

Check (✓) if normal, _NE_ if not examined, and _X_ if abnormal. Describe abnormal findings.

Description

_____ Vulva: No inflammation or edema

_____ No tenderness or masses

_____ Vaginal outlet: Good muscle tone, no bulging of mucosa

_____ Vagina: Mucosa pink, moist

_____ No lesions

_____ No excessive discharge

_____ Urethra: No inflammation or discharge

_____ Cervix: Position normal

_____ No lesions, nodules, or ulcerations

_____ No bleeding or discharge

_____ Uterus: Anterior, midline

_____ Smooth

_____ Not enlarged

_____ Adnexal: Ovaries normal size and consistency

_____ Nontender

_____ Rectovaginal exam: No masses

_____ Pap smear

Geriatric Adaptations— Physical

_____ Scanty pubic hair

_____ External genitalia atrophied

_____ Vaginal outlet: Weakened muscle tone

_____ No bulging of mucosa (observe for cystocele and rectocele)

_____ No leukoplakia

_____ Vaginal mucosa pale, thin

_____ Scanty amount of vaginal discharge

_____ Uterus small

_____ No prolapse of uterus

_____ Ovaries nonpalpable

Pediatric Adaptions— Physical

Infant/Child

_____ Absence of pubic hair

_____ No fusion of labia minora

_____ No vaginal discharge

Preadolescent/Adolescent

_____ Presence of pubic hair

_____ Presence of vaginal discharge

Disposition, recommendations, or treatment of abnormal findings:

Student_____

INSTRUCTOR'S GUIDE FOR EVALUATION OF STUDENT PERFOR-MANCE

Assessment of the Female Genitalia, Part 1

Behaviors evaluated	Yes	No	Remarks
1. Assembles equipment needed			
2. Explains procedure to client			
3. Places client in lithotomy position			
4. Drapes client to expose only area being examined			
5. Inspects external genitalia for			
a. Inflammation			
b. Lesions			
c. Discharge			
d. Distribution of pubic hair			
e. Bulging of vaginal walls when client strains down			
6. Palpates the Bartholin's glands by compressing posterior labia majora between index finger and thumb			
7. Uses water for lubrication if cytological examination is to be done			
8. Inserts vaginal speculum in oblique position, then rotates to horizontal position			
9. Inspects cervix for			
a. Position			
b. Ulcerations			
c. Nodules			
d. Masses			
e. Bleeding			
f. Discharge			
10. Obtains specimen for cytology exam from			
a. Endocervix (swab)			
b. Cervix (scrape)			
c. Vaginal pool, or (if cervix removed) from			
(1) Vaginal pool			
(2) Vaginal cuff			

Behaviors evaluated	Yes	No	Remarks
11. Observes vagina for			
a. Color of mucosa			
b. Inflammation			
c. Discharge			
d. Ulcers			
e. Masses			
12. Performs bimanual examination of uterus and adnexa and assesses			
a. Size			
b. Shape			
c. Consistency			
d. Mobility			
e. Tenderness			
13. Records all assessment findings using appropriate terminology			

Instructor _____ Date _____

MODULE 14

ASSESSMENT OF THE FEMALE GENITALIA, PART 2, ADAPTATIONS FOR THE OBSTETRICAL CLIENT

This instructional module is designed as a guide to assist you in learning a systematic approach for obtaining a health history and making an assessment of the genitalia of the obstetrical client. Section 14-1 (external genitalia) focuses upon observation of the perineum during the intrapartal period, while Sec. 14-3 (external genitalia) emphasizes assessment of the perineum during the immediate postpartal period. Section 14-2 (internal genitalia) is intended for the advanced nurse practitioner or nurse-midwife who assumes responsibility for determination of internal pelvic measurements, confirmation of pregnancy, assessment of fetopelvic relationships, and progress of labor.

This module can be completed most effectively in the obstetrical care setting as opposed to a learning laboratory. Information gained from Secs. 14-1 and 14-2 can best be utilized to help determine labor progress when utilized in combination with assessment data from Module 10 (assessment of the abdomen of the obstetrical client). Utilization of Sec. 14-3 of this module (observation of the perineum of the postpartal client) will be most effective in combination with Module 10, Part 2 (material regarding the fundal check of the abdomen of the obstetrical client) for the purpose of determining the recovery process of the puerperal client.

The format of this module is similar to previous modules. You are to complete this module and pass the Posttest before the scheduled practicum for assessment of the obstetrical client.

TERMINAL
OBJECTIVES

Upon completion of this module you are expected to be able to:

Sec. 14-1
(Observation of the perineum during the intrapartal period)

1. State the significance of assessment of the perineum throughout the intrapartal period.
2. Describe the characteristics of show.
3. Differentiate between show and bleeding.
4. Describe the characteristics of amniotic fluid.
5. State the purpose of the phenaphthazine (Nitrazine) test.
6. Define *bulging.*
7. Define *crowning.*
8. Define *episiotomy.*

Sec. 14-2
(Assessment of internal genitalia: prenatal and intrapartal periods)

1. State the expected findings to be obtained when examining the client to validate a pregnancy.
2. Describe the utilization of findings from a bimanual examination in determination of estimated date of confinement.
3. State the obstetrical significance of assessment of pelvic measurements in the prenatal and intrapartal periods.
4. Define *clinical pelvimetry.*
5. State the average measurements of the pelvic inlet, the midpelvis and the pelvic outlet.
6. Name the four classic types of pelves.
7. State the purpose of x-ray pelvimetry.
8. State the relationship of the fetal head to the maternal pelvis.
9. State what information about fetal lie, position, and presentation may be obtained from a pelvic examination.
10. Explain how the progress of labor may be determined through pelvic assessment.
11. State what precautions need to be taken when performing a pelvic examination on a pregnant woman.
12. Perform an assessment of the internal genitalia, collecting data on pregnancy confirmation, pelvic measurements, fetopelvic relationships, and progress of labor.

Section 14-3
(Observation of the perineum in the immediate postpartal period)

1. State three signs of placental separation occurring after the birth of the baby.
2. Define *lochia* and describe its characteristic changes during the puerperium.

SUGGESTED ACTIVITIES

Read

Ziegel, Erna E., and Mecca Cranley: "Antepartum Care — Data Collection and Assessment," "Obstetric Anatomy of Mother and Baby — The Passage and the Passenger," "Presentation and Position of the Fetus," "The Clinical Course and Mechanism of Labor and Delivery — Vaginal Examination by the Nurse," and "Clinical Management During Delivery — Immediate Post-Partum Period," *Obstetrical Nursing,* Macmillan, New York, 1978.

OR

Jensen, Margaret Duncan, et al.: "Management of the Antepartal Period," "Diagnosis of Pregnancy, Antepartal Examination Procedures," "Normal Labor," "First Stage of Labor," "Second Stage of Labor," and "Third and Fourth Stages of Labor," *Maternity Care: The Nurse and the Family,* Mosby, St. Louis, 1977.

View

Anatomy of the Female Pelvis and Reproductive Organs, Medical Electronic Educational Services filmstrip (MN-01).

Feto-Pelvic Relationships, Medical Electronic Educational Services filmstrip (MN-05).

Observing Contractions, Medical Electronic Educational Services filmstrip (LD-03).

Observing Fetal Heart Tones, Medical Electronic Educational Services filmstrip (LD-04).

Educational Aid

Obstetrical Presentation and Position, Ross Clinical Educational Aid No. 13.

Equipment

sterile glove

sterile lubricating jelly

VOCABULARY

Sec. 14-1

amniotic fluid	crowning	Nitrazine test
bulging	episiotomy	show

Sec. 14-2

android	fontanels	pelvic inlet
anthropoid	gynecoid	pelvimetry
bregma	Hegar's sign	pelvic outlet
Chadwick's sign	ischial spine	platypelloid
diagonal conjugate	midpelvis	sinciput
dilatation	molding	suboccipito bregmatic
effacement	obstetric conjugate	sutures
engagement	occipitofrontal diameter	true pelvis
false pelvis	occiput	vertex

Sec. 14-3

alba	lochia	rubra	serosa

DECISION TABLE 14-1

If . . .		Then . . .
You need additional information on confirmation of pregnancy	⟹	MacDonald, Paul C., and Jack A. Pritchard: "Diagnosis of Pregnancy," *Williams Obstetrics*, 5th ed., Appleton-Century-Crofts, New York, 1976.
You wish to do additional reading on pelvic anatomy from an obstetric point of view	⟹	MacDonald, Paul C., and Jack A. Pritchard: "The Normal Pelvis," *Williams Obstetrics*, 5th ed., Appleton-Century-Crofts, New York, 1976.
You still need assistance understanding presentation, position, and lie of the fetus	⟹	MacDonald, Paul C., and Jack A. Pritchard: "Presentation, Position, Attitude, and Lie of Fetus," *Williams Obstetrics*, 5th ed., Appleton-Century-Crofts, New York, 1976.
	⟹	Oxorn, Harry, and William R. Foote: "Obstetric Pelvis," "The Passenger: Fetus," and "Fetopelvic Relationships," *Human Labor and Birth*, Appleton-Century-Crofts, New York, 1975.
You wish to review a systematic approach to examination of the obstetrical client	⟹	Oxorn, Harry, and William R. Foote: "Examination of the Patient," *Human Labor and Birth*, Appleton-Century-Crofts, New York, 1975.
You want to extend your knowledge to include screening for high-risk obstetrical clients	⟹	Blair, Carole Lotito, and Elizabeth Meehan Salerno: "Screening Tool for High Risk Clients," *The Expanding Family: Childbearing*, Little, Brown, Boston, 1976.
You wish to prepare yourself to care for clients from various sociocultural groups	⟹	Blair, Carole Lotito, and Elizabeth Meehan Salerno: "Sociocultural Index of Childbearing," *The Expanding Family: Childbearing*, Little, Brown, Boston, 1976.

POSTTEST

Sec. 14-1 (external genitalia)

1. List *four* reasons for observation of the perineum throughout labor.

   a. _____

   b. _____

   c. _____

   d. _____

2. Describe the nature of *show*.

Write *true* or *false.* If *false,* correct the statement to make it true.

3. _____ Bloody show increases in amount as the cervix thins and dilates.
4. _____ A sudden and marked increase in bloody show is often indicative of the second stage of labor.
5. _____ A gush of bright red blood normally appears in midlabor.
6. _____ Normal amniotic fluid is watery and slightly greenish in color.
7. _____ A Nitrazine test reading of a pH below 6.0 is indicative of intact membranes.

8. Normal amniotic fluid
   a. Is odorless
   b. Has a sweet odor
   c. Has an odor like urine
9. Meconium-stained amniotic fluid is a sign of fetal distress except in what circumstances?

10. Bulging of the perineum in labor is a sign of _____.
11. Define *crowning.*

12. What is the significance of crowning?

13. Define *episiotomy.*

14. Explain the purpose of an episiotomy.

Sec. 14-2 (internal genitalia)

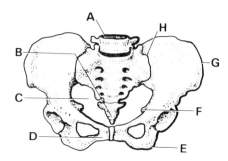

Figure 14-1

1. Label Fig. 14-1, which depicts the structure of the female pelvis.

   a.   e.

   b.   f.

   c.   g.

   d.   h.

2. Define *Hegar's sign.*

3. Define *Chadwick's sign.*

4. The function of the false pelvis is to _____.

5. The function of the true (lesser) pelvis is to _____

   _____.

6. The fetal head enters the birth canal at the _____.

7. Label the three diameters of the pelvic inlet below and state their diameters.

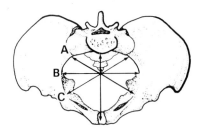

Figure 14-2

a. _____   _____

b. _____   _____

c. _____   _____

8. The _____ diameter is the shortest measurement of the pelvic inlet.

Write *true* or *false.* If *false,* correct the statement to make it true.

9. _____   The *true conjugate* is the distance from the top of the symphysis pubis to the middle of the promontory of the sacrum.

10. _____   The diagonal conjugate, the distance from the lower margin of the symphysis pubis to the sacral promontory, is the only diameter of the inlet which may be measured without use of x-ray.

11. _____   The most common form of pelvic inlet contraction is the inadequacy of the anterior-posterior diameter of the inlet (the obstetric conjugate).

12. Label Fig. 14-3. Then designate the average length of important diameters of the fetal skull.

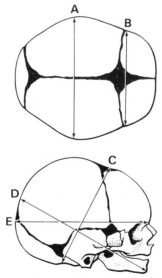

Figure 14-3

a. _____

b. _____

c. _____

d. _____

e. _____

13. Why are the fetal sutures and fontanels of diagnostic value during labor?

14. The fetal head usually enters the pelvis with the suboccipitobregmatic diameter lying parallel to the _____ diameter of the pelvic inlet.

15. The narrowest area of the birth canal, also referred to as the *plane of least pelvic dimensions,* is the _____.

16. The distance between the ischial spines is of obstetrical significance because

_____

_____

17. The smallest anterior-posterior diameter of the pelvis (midpelvis) is _____ cm.

18. The smallest transverse diameter of the pelvis (midpelvis) is _____ cm.

19. The fetal head emerges from the birth canal at the _____

_____ .

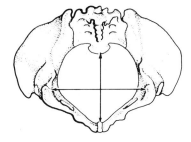

Figure 14-4

20. Label Fig. 14-4. Then designate the two important diameters of the pelvic outlet.

    a. The transverse diameter is _____ cm.

    b. The anterior-posterior diameter is _____ cm.

21. The *mechanism of labor* is defined as _____

_____ .

22. Name the *four* general classifications of pelves.

    a. _____   c. _____

    b. _____   d. _____

23. The inlet of the feminine pelvis is _____ shaped.

24. What is a *contracted pelvis?*

25. *Cervical effacement* is _____

_____ .

26. To ascertain the amount of effacement by pelvic examination, the cervix is pal-

pated for _____

and _____ .

27. *Cervical dilatation* is _____

_____ .

28. To measure cervical dilatation by pelvic examination, an estimate is made of

_____ .

29. The descent (station) of the fetal head is measured in relationship to the

_____ .

30. The station of the fetal head is stated in _____ terms.

31. Explain the significance of the following fetal stations:

a. − 1 _____

b.   0 _____

c. + 1 _____

32. When combined abdominal and pelvic palpation reveals the presenting part to be

freely movable above the pelvic inlet, it is described as _____ .

33. When the fetal presenting part is no longer movable, it is said to be _____

_____ .

34. Engagement of the fetal head is _____

_____ .

Sec. 14-3

1. Describe *two* observations of the perineum immediately following delivery which
are indicative of placental separation.

a. _____

b. _____

2. Name *three* types of lochia and describe their appearance.

   a. _____

   b. _____

   c. _____

3. State the approximate day postdelivery on which the following types of lochia occur.

   a. _____ Rubra

   b. _____ Serosa

   c. _____ Alba

HEALTH HISTORY AND ASSESSMENT

This information should be obtained from the pregnant client in addition to a general health history which includes client identifying data, previous medical history, family medical history, and socioeconomic and cultural history (Module 1).

History of Obstetrical Client Pertinent to Assessment of the Female Genitalia

Remarks

1. First day of last menstrual period?
2. Pregnancy planned or unplanned?
3. If pregnancy unplanned, type of contraception at time of conception?
4. Previous menstrual period (first day of period before last menstrual period)?
5. Interval of usual menstrual cycle?
6. Number of previous pregnancies?
7. Number of miscarriages (abortions)?
8. Number of full-term births (9 months)?
9. Number of premature births (less than 8½ months)?
10. Number of living children?
11. Number of multiple births (twins, triplets)?
12. Complications of previous pregnancies (nausea and vomiting, bleeding, toxemia)?
13. Use of
    a. Tobacco (number of cigarettes per day)
    b. Alcohol (amount and kind of beverages consumed daily)
    c. Soft or hard drugs (LSD, marijuana, heroin)
    d. Prescription or nonprescription drugs
14. X-ray examination within past 6 months?
15. Illnesses and their treatment since last menstrual period?
16. Exposure to individuals with illnesses since last menstrual period?

17. Method of previous deliveries (vaginal or cesarean section)?
18. Length of previous labors?
19. Complications of previous labors or deliveries?
20. Anesthetics with previous labors or deliveries?
21. Weight of previously delivered infants?

Information about father of baby
1. Age?
2. Height?
3. Weight?
4. Blood type?
5. Any blood relationship of father and mother?
   Yes _____   No _____
6. Chronic or acute health problems?

Additional information to be obtained if client in labor
1. Childbirth education?
2. Type of analgesia or anesthetic planned?
3. Lightening (patient's subjective report)?
   When occurred? _____
4. Show? Yes _____ No _____
5. Membranes
   Intact? _____
   Ruptured? _____
   Date? _____ Time? _____
6. Onset of contractions?
7. Time contractions became regular?
8. Last food intake (time, date, kind of food)?
9. Last time patient slept?
10. Last voiding?
11. Last defecation?

Additional information to be obtained if client has delivered

1. Length of time since delivery?
2. Complications of delivery?
3. Method of placental delivery?*

    Manual _____ Spontaneous _____
4. Weight of infant?
5. Oxytocic drugs received (dosage, frequency)?*
6. Fundal height, shape, and consistency immediately following delivery?*

*Information may be obtained from client's medical record.

Physical Assessment of the Female Genitalia: Adaptations for the Obstetrical Client

Check (✓) if present or fill in the blanks as appropriate.

Prenatal assessment   Description

External genitalia

_____ Distribution of pubic hair

_____ Lesions

_____ Warts

_____ Discharge from vagina: Color, odor, consistency, irritation of surrounding skin

_____ Perineal support or degree of relaxation

_____ Varicosities

Internal genitalia

_____ Vagina: Color (Chadwick's sign), mucosa

_____ Cervix: Consistency (Goodell's sign), color, position (anterior, posterior), scars

_____ Isthmus: Consistency (Hegar's sign)

_____ Uterus: Shape, size (assessment of enlargement), position (anterior, retroverted), mobility

Pelvic capacity

_____ Inlet:

    _____ Anterior-posterior diameter

    _____ Transverse diameter

    Midpelvis:

    _____ Anterior-posterior diameter,

    _____ Transverse diameter

    _____ Prominence of ischial spines

_____ Outlet:

    Anterior-posterior diameter, transverse diameter, mobility of coccyx

_____ Summary of pelvic capacity

    _____Adequate

    _____Inadequate (describe)

    _____Borderline (describe)

Intrapartal assessment

External genitalia

_____ Lesions

_____ Warts

_____ Varicosities

_____ Show (describe)

_____ Presence of amniotic fluid, color, odor, amount

_____ Flattening of perineum

_____ Bulging

_____ Crowning

_____ External prolapse of umbilical cord

Internal genitalia

_____ Reassessment of pelvic capacity

_____ Adequate

_____ Inadequate

Cervix: Effacement, dilatation (Describe.)

Assessment of degree (station) of fetal descent (state phase of labor) (Describe.)

Lie of fetus (state phase of labor) (Describe.)

_____ Presentation of fetus (state phase of labor)

_____ Position of fetus (state phase of labor); describe identification of fetal head suture lines if cephalic presentation

Immediate postdelivery

External genitalia

Third stage of labor

_____ Visual lengthening of umbilical cord protruding from vagina

_____ Gush of bright red blood

Fourth stage of labor

_____ Lochia

Type

Amount

Clots

Swelling of perineum

Hematoma formation

Student_____

INSTRUCTOR'S GUIDE FOR EVALUATION OF STUDENT PERFOR-MANCE

Assessment of female genitalia: obstetrical client

Behaviors evaluated	Yes	No	Remarks
1. Assembles equipment needed			
2. Takes appropriate history for genitalia of the obstetrical client			
3. Explains procedure to client			
4. Places client in lithotomy position			
5. Drapes to expose genitalia only			
6. Inspects external genitalia as appropriate prenatally, intrapartally, or postpartally			
Prenatally			
a. Inspects skin for lesions or warts			
b. Assesses vaginal introitus for discharge			
Intrapartally			
a. Inspects skin for lesions, warts, discharge, varicosities			
b. Inspects perineum for show — amount, color, consistency			
c. Inspects perineum for presence of amniotic fluid — amount, color, odor			
d. Inspects perineum for presence of externally prolapsed umbilical cord			
e. Inspects perineum for flattening, bulging, crowning			
Postpartally			
Third stage of labor			
a. Inspects perineum for visible lengthening of umbilical cord protruding from vagina			
b. Inspects perineum for gush of bright red blood			
Fourth stage of labor			
a. Inspects perineum for lochia — type, amount, clots			
b. Inspects perineum for swelling or hematoma formation			

Behaviors evaluated	Yes	No	Remarks
7. Inspects internal genitalia			
Prenatally			
a. Vagina color, mucosa			
b. Cervix—Goodell's sign, color, position, scars			
c. Isthmus—Hegar's sign			
d. Uterus—shape, size, position, mobility			
e. Pelvic capacity—inlet, midpelvis, outlet			
Intrapartally			
a. Reassesses pelvic capacity			
b. Assesses cervical effacement, dilatation			
c. Assesses degree of fetal descent			
d. Assesses presentation of fetus			
e. Assesses lie of fetus			
f. Assesses position of fetus			

Instructor _____ Date _____

MODULE 15

ASSESSMENT OF THE MUSCULOSKELETAL SYSTEM

Mobility and performance of the activities of daily living are key elements in human self-esteem and depend upon smooth functioning of the musculoskeletal system. This module is designed to assist you in performing a thorough and systematic assessment of the musculoskeletal system. Assessment of both structure and function is primarily achieved through use of the inspection and palpation techniques. Both the history and the physical examination should be utilized to achieve a thorough assessment of the client's ability to perform the activities of daily living. In addition, emphasis will be placed on observation of gait, symmetry of joints, muscles and bones, and range of motion.

The format of this module is similar to previous modules. You are to complete this module and pass the Posttest before the scheduled practicum for assessment of the musculoskeletal system.

If you have questions, contact your instructor.

PREREQUISITE OBJECTIVES

You should be able to:

1. Label the anatomical structures on a diagram of the human musculoskeletal system.
2. Label the anatomical structures on a diagram of a joint.
3. Describe the functions of joints and their structures.
4. Describe the normal spinal curvatures of infants and adults.
5. Describe posture and identify body functions which are affected by posture.

TERMINAL OBJECTIVES

Upon completion of this module you are expected to be able to:

1. Define the vocabulary words accompanying this module.
2. Given an assessment form as a guide, take a complete health history pertinent to the musculoskeletal system using appropriate branching questions.
3. Describe the existing anatomical differences between the musculoskeletal system of the infant, child, and adult that will be of significance to the examiner.
4. Discuss the use of the Denver Developmental Screening Test in assessing the musculoskeletal system of children.
5. Describe the effect of the "growth spurt" on skeletal development.
6. Describe structural and functional changes in the musculoskeletal system that occur with aging.
7. Describe variations in physical findings among ethnic groups.
8. Demonstrate evaluation of ability to perform activities of daily living.
9. Discuss the five factors used to assess gait:

    stance

    swing

    balance

    step size

    arm swing and need to watch feet

10. Demonstrate assessment of gait.
11. Describe a client's gait.
12. Demonstrate assessment of body symmetry.
13. Demonstrate assessment of body posture.
14. Demonstrate assessment of spinal curvatures and identify abnormalities.
15. Demonstrate assessment of muscle strength and tone in each extremity.
16. Demonstrate assessment of range of motion for each joint.
17. Palpate muscles and joints for tenderness, swelling, and symmetry.
18. Test joints for crepitation.
19. Demonstrate evaluation for congenital dislocation of the hip and tibial torsion.
20. Demonstrate assessment of knee for torn meniscus and for stability.
21. Demonstrate assessment for sciatica.
22. Record the data obtained from the health assessment using correct medical terminology.

SUGGESTED ACTIVITIES

Read

Alexander, M. M., and M. S. Brown: "Physical Examination, Part 16: The Musculoskeletal System," *Nursing '76,* 51–56 (April, 1976).

OR

Alexander, Mary M. and Marie Scott Brown: "The Skeletal System: Spine and Extremities," *Pediatric History Taking and Physical Diagnosis for Nurses,* McGraw-Hill, New York, 1979.

Bates, Barbara: *A Guide to Physical Assessment,* Lippincott, Philadelphia, 1979.

OR

Malasanos, Lois, et al.: "Musculoskeletal Assessment," *Health Assessment,* Mosby, St. Louis, 1977.

Caird, F. I., and T. G. Judge: *Assessment of the Elderly Patient,* Pitman, Calif., 1977.

OR

Saxon, Sue V., and Mary Jean Etten: *Physical Change and Aging,* The Tiresias Press, New York, 1978.

DeGowin, Elmer L., and Richard L. DeGowin: "Motor Functions—The Gait," *Diagnostic Examination,* 3d ed., 1976.

Murray, Ruth B., and Judith Zentner: *Nursing Assessment and Health Promotion Through the Life Span,* Prentice-Hall, Englewood Cliffs, N.J., 1979, pp. 162–164, 211.

View

Bates, Barbara: *Examination of the Musculoskeletal System,* Lippincott videotape, 30 min.

Pediatric Physical Examination: The Skeletal Sytem, Blue Hill Educational Systems, 25 min.

Physical Assessment Examinations: Musculoskeletal, Blue Hill Educational Systems videotape, 18 min.

Equipment

    goniometer (if desired)

    centimeter measuring tape (plastic)

If neurological screening is included:

    reflex hammer

    penlight

    two test tubes (one filled with hot water and one filled with cold water)

    tuning fork

    safety pins (2)

PRETEST   1. On Fig. 15-1, label the bones and joints indicated by the arrows.

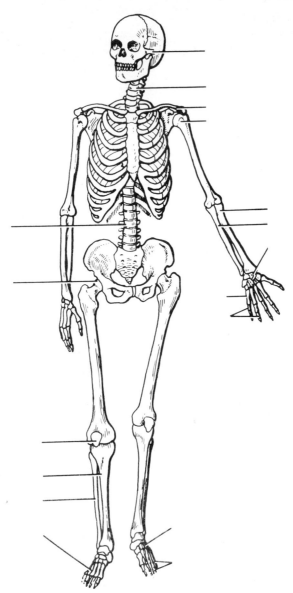

Figure 15-1

2. On Figs. 15-2 and 15-3, label the muscles indicated by arrows.

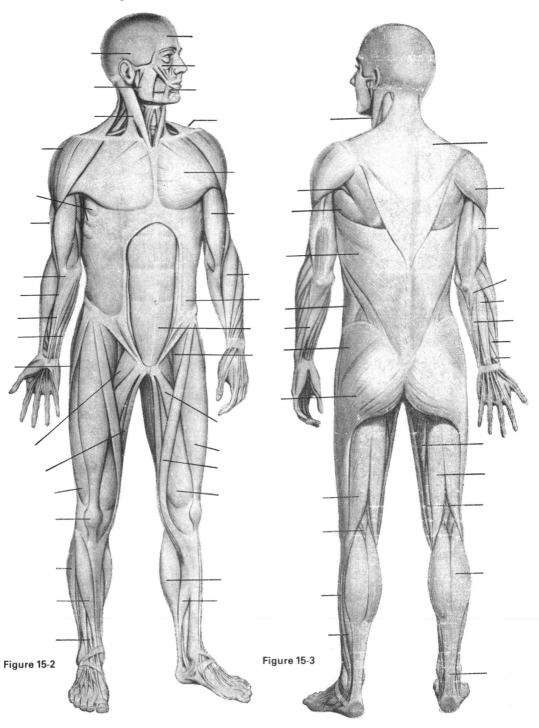

Figure 15-2   **Figure 15-3**

3. Label the joint structures on Fig. 15-4.

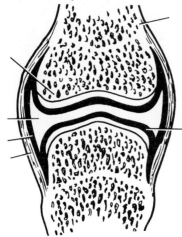

Figure 15-4

4. The purpose of articular cartilage in a joint is to provide a _____

   between the _____ .

5. A _____ is a disk-shaped fluid-filled
   synovial sac that facilitates motion and decreases friction.

6. Draw and label the normal spinal curvatures.

7. Which of these curves are not present at birth?

8. Which of the following joints are diarthrosis joints?
   a. 1, 2, 4, 5   1. Knee
   b. 1, 3, 4, 5   2. Vertebral
   c. 2, 4 only   3. Temporomandibular
   d. 1, 3, 5 only   4. Elbow
   e. All   5. Shoulder
9. What is the importance of the epiphysis?

10. Which of the following functions are affected by posture?

a. 1, 2, 4	1. Joint action
b. 2, 3, 5	2. Memory
c. All except 2	3. Respiration
d. 3, 4, 5	4. Circulation
e. All except 1	5. Digestion

11. Weak places in the abdominal wall include

a. 1, 2, 3	1. Femoral ring
b. 2, 3, 5	2. Inguinal ring
c. 3, 4, 5	3. Symphysis pubis
d. 1, 2, 5	4. Umbilicus
e. 1, 2, 4	5. Linea negra

VOCABULARY   Descriptive terminology

abduction	gait:	plantar
adduction	ataxic	plantar flexion
ankylosis	parkinsonian	pronation
ataxia	scissor	radial deviation
bursa	shuffling	range of motion (ROM)
circumduction	spastic	rotation (external and internal)
concave	staggering	scoliosis
contracture	waddling	steppage
convex	ganglion	subluxation
crepitation	hyperextension	supination
dorsal	inversion	"swan-neck" deformity
dorsiflex	kyphosis	tibial torsion
eversion	lordosis	tic
extension	meningocele	tone
fasciculation	nodule	tonic
flexion	olecranon process	tremor
	pilonidal cyst	ulnar deviation

Diagnostic terminology

ankylosing spondylitis	Homan's sign	pes varus
Dupuytren's contracture	metatarsus valgus	rheumatoid arthritis
genu valgum	metatarsus varus	sciatica
genu varum	Ortolani's test	talipes equinovarus
growth spurt	osteoarthritis	torticollis
hallus valgus	pes planus	Trendelenburg's sign
Heberden's node	pes valgus	

DECISION TABLE 15-1

If . . .   **Then . . .**

You need help with pediatric inter-   ⟹   Chinn, Peggy L. and Cynthia Leitch:
viewing for the health history   *Child Health Maintenance: A Guide
                                              to Clinical Assessment,* Mosby, St.
                                              Louis, 2nd ed., 1979.

You need help in evaluating activities ⟹   Coley, Ida Lou: *Pediatric Assess-
of daily living   ment of Self-Care Activities,* Mosby,
                                              St. Louis, 1978.

You prefer color photographs of   ⟹   Mead Johnson Company: *The Ex-
variations of extremities in the   tremities — Parts 1 and 2,* Evansville,
newborn infant   Ind.

You seek additional or alternative   ⟹   *Pediatric Physical Examination — The
media   Neuromuscular System — School Age
                                              Child,* Blue Hill Educational Systems,
                                              50 min; *Infant,* 29 min.

You want more information on   ⟹   Erickson, Marcene: *Assessment and
assessment and management of   Management of Developmental
growth and developmental delays   Changes in Children,* Mosby, St.
                                              Louis, 1976.

POSTTEST

1. A *swan-neck deformity* refers to a deformity of the _____ .

2. Leg length is measured from the _____ _____

   to the _____ with the client in the _____

   position.

3. Ortolani's test is performed to check for _____ .

4. *Ankylosis* is defined as _____ .

5. If spondylitis is present, check chest _____ .

6. Describe a method of detecting fluid in the knee.

   _____

   _____

7. The hands and wrists are inspected for

   a. _____

   b. _____

   c. _____

d. _____

e. _____

8. Joints are checked for

   a. _____

   b. _____

   c. _____

   d. _____

9. Match the terms in the left column with the definitions in the right column.

   a. Concave   _____ An incomplete dislocation or displacement
   b. Pes valgus   _____ Soft, flabby, relaxed
   c. Torticollis   _____ An acquired local reduction in size of a tissue or body
   d. Flaccid   part
   e. Pes planus   _____ Grating sound, crackling
   f. Kyphosis   _____ Flat feet
   g. Subluxation   _____ Contraction deformity of cervical muscles
   h. Convex   _____ Forward curvature of lumbar spine
   i. Lordosis   _____ An outward swelling or rounding of an external
   j. Atrophy   surface
   k. Crepitation

10. Radial deviation of the wrist is (*greater than, less than*) ulnar deviation.

11. Heberden's nodes are (*normal, abnormal*) in a person over 55 years old.

12. When a client complains of pain in a joint, what information should be elicited about the pain?

    a. _____

    b. _____

    c. _____

    d. _____

13. The description of a client's gait should include:

    a. _____

    b. _____

    c. _____

    d. _____

    e. _____

    f. _____

14. Describe the gait of a client with paralysis of the dorsiflexors of one foot.

Write *true* or *false.* If *false,* correct the statement to make it true.

15. _____ Fracture of the clavicles is one of the most common injuries to the infant at birth.

16. _____ A child between the ages of 2 and 3½ should be referred for evaluation if genu varum exists.

17. _____ A child of 12 months should be referred when flat feet are observed.

18. _____ When examining the infant, dislocation of the hip should be suspected if a click is heard and the femur slips out of the acetabulum.

19. _____ Functional scoliosis will disappear when the child flexes spine 60°. This type of scoliosis does not require referral.

20. _____ Positional deformities of the infant's foot cannot be corrected to the neutral position.

21. _____ A child of 2½ should be referred if unable to balance when standing on one foot for 10 seconds.

22. _____ A 12-month-old boy should be referred because he topples over when stooping to recover objects.

23. _____ A young man who reports no growth spurt by age 14 needs to be referred.

24. _____ During the period of the growth spurt, a girl may grow as much as 5 in.

HEALTH HISTORY AND ASSESSMENT

If the answer is yes, place a check (✔) at the left and provide further information in the Remarks column.

Remarks

Adult Health History: Musculoskeletal System

_____ Poor coordination of movements?

_____ Swollen or painful joints?

_____ Decreased range of motion?

_____ Stiffness of muscles or joints?

_____ Painful feet, hands?

_____ Backache?

_____ Pain or stiffness in neck?

_____ Sprain or fracture?

_____ Muscle weakness?

_____ Muscle twitching?

_____ Muscle cramps in arms or legs?

_____ Difficulty with combing hair, feeding self, brushing teeth, bathing and dressing self, turning pages in a book, holding a pen?

_____ Difficulty in sitting, standing, lying down, walking, sitting up or getting up, climbing, pinching, grasping, leaning over?

Geriatric Adaptations— History

_____ Recent fall?

_____ Morning stiffness of joints?

_____ Difficulty getting out of chair?

_____ Use a cane or walker?

_____ Difficulty going up or down stairs?

_____ Difficulty picking up objects?

_____ History of arthritis, bursitis, gout, fractures, paralysis?

_____ Description of daily activity or exercise pattern _____

_____

Pediatric Adaptations— History

_____ Age child began walking? ____
_____ History of birth injury?
_____ Sits in "TV squat" (position with knees and ankles flexed and flat on floor to the side and extended behind)?
_____ Wears down shoes unevenly? More on one side than another?
_____ Participate in athletic activities? Describe _____
_____ Limitation of movement in extremities?
_____ Pain in muscles, joints, or extremities?
_____ Diet adequate in vitamin C, D, calcium?
_____ History of trauma to bones, joints, muscles?

Adult Physical Assessment— Musculo- skeletal System

Check (✓) if normal, _NE_ if not examined, _X_ if abnormal. Describe abnormal findings.

Head and Neck   Description
_____ Full ROM of eyes
_____ No deformities
_____ Facial muscle strength normal, symmetrical
_____ No abnormal posture
_____ Full ROM temperomandibular joint
_____ No crepitus, tenderness, swell- ing/fluid, or bony enlargement
_____ Full ROM of cervical spine
_____ No deformity, redness, swell- ing, nodules, or muscle atrophy
_____ Normal muscle strength in head and neck

Shoulders and arms
_____ Full ROM of shoulders
_____ Shoulders level

_____ No swelling, redness, nodules, or bony enlargement

_____ Equal arm circumferences and lengths

_____ No deformity or atrophy

_____ Muscle strength normal, symmetrical

_____ Full ROM of elbows

_____ No joint deformity, swelling/ fluid, bony enlargement, tenderness

_____ Normal muscle strength

Hands and wrists

_____ Full ROM

_____ No swelling/fluid, deformity, atrophy, or bony enlargement

_____ No tenderness or crepitation

_____ Normal muscle strength

Thorax

_____ Costochondral junctions: No swelling or tenderness

_____ No rosary beads

_____ Rib cage symmetrical

_____ Clearly defined intercostal spaces

_____ Ribs intact

_____ Clavicles intact (not unduly prominent or sunken)

_____ Sternum smooth (not depressed or protuberant)

_____ Ribs slope downward at 45° angle

_____ No bone crepitus

Hips and knees

_____ Full ROM

_____ Normal muscle strength

_____ No deformity, crepitus, fluid, tenderness, atrophy, or bony enlargement

_____ Leg and hip-to-knee lengths
are equal

_____ Muscle circumferences are
equal

_____ No crepitus

Feet and ankles

_____ Full ROM

_____ No deformities or nodules

_____ No calluses, corns, or bony
enlargement

_____ No tenderness or swelling/fluid

_____ Normal muscle strength

_____ No crepitus

Spine

_____ Body alignment/posture

_____ No scoliosis, lordosis, or
kyphosis

_____ No tenderness or spasms of
paravertebral and trapezius
muscles

_____ No tenderness of spine

_____ Full ROM

_____ No pain on straight-leg lifting

Reflexes*

_____ Biceps reflex

_____ Triceps reflex

_____ Brachioradialis reflex

_____ Patellar reflex

_____ Achilles reflex

_____ Plantar reflex

_____ Cremasteric reflex

_____ Gluteal reflex

_____ Grasp reflex

*Reflexes are a part of the neurological examination, but pertinent to the musculoskeletal exam.

Activities of daily living

_____ Sits down

_____ Lies down

_____ Sits up

_____ Gets up

_____ Stands

_____ Walks/gait

_____ Bends over and retrieves objects

_____ Ties shoes

Geriatric Adaptations— Physical

_____ Mild scoliosis

_____ Mild kyphosis

_____ Stooped body posture

_____ Diminished muscle strength bilaterally

_____ Diminished muscle mass

_____ Diminished joint flexibility

Pediatric Adaptations— Physical

_____ Results on fine and gross motor sectors of DDST are within normal limits for age

_____ Genu varum is frequently seen in infants until they have been walking for 1 year

_____ Infants: Bilateral hip rotation of 160 to 175°

_____ Infants with protruding abdomens will have slight degree of lumbar lordosis

_____ Thoracic curve of spine present in newborn

_____ Infant: At rest may hold position in utero

_____ Infant: Positional deformity of foot can be manipulated to neutral position

_____ Genu valgum may be present
between 2 and 3½ years

_____ Ortolani's sign absent

_____ No metatarsus varus or metatarsus valgus

_____ No tibial torsion past age 2

_____ Lumbar curve present if child
is walking

_____ No absence of body parts or
presence of extra body parts

_____ No shortening/lengthening of
extremities

_____ Posture straight and erect

_____ No pilonidal cyst/meningocele

_____ Trendelenburg's sign absent

_____ Growth spurt in preadoles-
cence or adolescence (girls
average 2½ to 5 in; boys average 3 to 6 in)

_____ Growth spurt proceeds se-
quentially (hands and feet,
calves and forearms, hips,
chest, shoulders, trunk)

By age 6

_____ Can walk chalk mark with
balance

_____ Can balance on one foot 10
seconds

_____ Can throw and catch a ball

_____ Can kick a ball

_____ Can walk forward heel to toe

_____ Can walk backward heel to toe

_____ Can pedal tricycle or bicycle

_____ Can cut with scissors

_____ Can copy geometric figures
with pencil

_____ Gait narrow-based

_____ Can skip

Ethnic Adaptations— Physical

_____ At age 2: Black child may be taller and heavier than white counterpart—will have greater skeletal development

_____ Skeletal mass greater in black client

_____ Black boys and girls attain a greater portion of adult height earlier than Caucasian youth

_____ Oriental and Latin individuals may show an earlier growth spurt and advanced maturity when compared to individuals of European extraction

_____ Mild lordosis may be present in black clients

Recommendations, treatment, or disposition of abnormal findings:

Student_____

INSTRUCTOR'S GUIDE FOR EVALUATION OF STUDENT PERFOR-MANCE

Assessment of the Musculoskeletal System

Behaviors evaluated	Yes	No	Remarks
1. Assembles equipment			
2. Takes appropriate history of musculo-skeletal system			
3. Asks branching questions when indicated			
4. Explains procedure for examination to client			
5. Provides adequate lighting			
6. Washes hands			
7. Compares right to left in each phase of the examination			
8. Assesses client's ability to perform activities of daily living: a. Sit, lie down, sit up, get up, stand, walk, grasp, bend over b. Comb hair, brush teeth, bathe and dress, feed self			
9. Inspects head and neck for deformities and abnormal posture			
10. Palpates both temperomandibular joints anterior to tragus, noting range of motion, crepitus, tenderness, or swelling			
11. Palpates cervical spine and neck muscles for tenderness			
12. Visually inspects body for symmetry, contour, and size of each side of the body			
13. Notes gross deformities, areas of swelling or edema, and areas of discoloration			
14. With client standing, checks posture and body alignment from in front of and from behind the client			
15. Spinal curvatures are noted			
16. From behind asks client to bend at waist; notes any deviation or deformity of spine			
17. With client lying down, the arms, upper arms, and forearms are compared for symmetry			

Behaviors evaluated	Yes	No	Remarks
18. Length of legs, thighs, and lower legs are compared for symmetry			
19. Maximum circumference of each limb can be used for comparison, especially when swelling or atrophy are suspected			
20. Checks ocular muscle strength by asking client to close eyes against resistance			
21. Checks range of motion of eye and notes appropriate tracking and lid lag			
22. Assesses facial muscles by asking client to blow out cheeks, notes pressure against fingers held against resultant cheek bulge			
23. Checks neck strength by asking client to bend head backward and then forward against resistance			
24. Deltoid muscle strength is checked by having client hold arms up against resistance and then keep arms extended while examiner tries to push them down			
25. Biceps muscle strength is checked by asking client to extend arms and then try to flex them against examiner resistance			
26. Triceps muscle strength is examined by asking client to flex arm and then extend it against examiner resistance			
27. Muscle strength in wrists and fingers is checked by asking client to extend hand and then to resist examiner's attempt to flex the wrist first with the client's fingers out and then with fingers together			
28. Hip strength is assessed by asking client to assume supine position and to raise extended legs alternately against resistance			
29. Hamstring, gluteal, abductor, and adductor leg muscle strength is assessed by asking client to sit and perform alternate leg crossing			
30. Quadricep muscle strength is assessed by asking client to extend leg stiffly while examiner tries to bend it			

Behaviors evaluated	Yes	No	Remarks
31. Hamstring muscle strength is assessed by asking client to bend knees while examiner tries to straighten them			
32. Muscle strength in the ankle and foot are checked by asking client to exert upward foot pressure and then big-toe pressure against examiner resistance			
33. Each muscle mass is tapped sharply to detect muscle fasciculations			
34. Deep tendon reflexes are checked:*			
a. Biceps reflex			
b. Triceps reflex			
c. Brachioradialis reflex			
d. Patellar reflex			
e. Achilles tendon reflex			
f. Plantar reflex			
35. Superficial reflexes are checked:			
a. Cremasteric reflex			
b. Gluteal reflex			
c. Grasp reflex			
36. Inspects the following joints for redness, swelling, nodules, deformity, or muscle atrophy:			
a. Neck			
b. Shoulders and arms			
c. Elbows			
d. Wrists			
e. Hands and fingers			
f. Hips			
g. Knees			
h. Feet and toes			
i. Ankles			
j. Spine			
37. Palpates each joint listed above for tenderness, swelling, bogginess (fluid), or bony enlargement			

*If a neurological exam is performed in conjunction with the musculoskeletal examination, the deep tendon and superficial reflex examination need not be duplicated.

Behaviors evaluated	Yes	No	Remarks
38. Tests complete range of motion, both active and passive, in each joint listed above[†]			
39. Describes client's gait			
40. Records findings using appropriate terminology			

[†]Usually not performed unless history or screening examination indicate a possible muscular or neural dysfunction in the client.

Instructor _____ Date _____

MODULE 16

ASSESSMENT OF THE NEUROLOGICAL SYSTEM

This instructional module is designed as a guide to assist you in learning a thorough and systematic approach to neurological assessment. Adaptations for assessing the infant, child, and geriatric client are included. Several portions of this exam have already been covered in previous modules. In fact, much of this neurological exam is covered in a routine physical assessment as you elicit the history and examine the body by regions. However, a complete and systematic neurological examination is indicated when abnormal function of the nervous system is discovered on a regional or routine physical exam.

The neurological exam is usually divided into five categories: (1) cranial nerves, (2) motor system, (3) sensory system, (4) reflexes, and (5) mental status and speech.

Mental status is one of the most important aspects of the neurological examination and is evaluated throughout the exam. Your assessment of mental status begins the moment you see the client and continues throughout the examination. Questions regarding mental status should not be asked until you have established some rapport with the client. For that reason, it is included at the end of the exam rather than at the beginning.

The format of this module is similar to that of the previous modules. You are to complete this module and pass the Posttest before the scheduled laboratory period for assessment of the neurological system.

If you have difficulty, contact your instructor.

PREREQUISITE OBJECTIVES

You should be able to:

1. Describe the functions of the cerebellar system.
2. Explain a simple reflex and how it is elicited.
3. Differentiate between the physiology of sensory and motor neurons.
4. Describe the functions of the brain stem.
5. Describe the sections and the functions of the brain and spinal cord.
6. Describe the functions of each of the cranial nerves.
7. Describe the physiology of the spinal cord and spinal nerves.

TERMINAL OBJECTIVES

Upon completion of this module you are expected to be able to:

1. Define the vocabulary words accompanying this module.
2. Using an assessment form as a guide, take a complete health history pertinent to neurological assessment.
3. Describe the alterations in levels of consciousness.
4. Describe the five categories of the neurological exam.
5. Evaluate the 12 pairs of cranial nerves.
6. Demonstrate at least three tests of cerebellar function.
7. Demonstrate assessment of motor function, balance, and coordination.
8. Demonstrate assessment of gait and describe gait abnormalities.
9. Demonstrate evaluation of perception related to body position, point discrimination, and stereognosis.
10. Demonstrate the evaluation of sensory responses to pain, touch, heat, and cold.
11. Demonstrate evaluation of superficial reflexes.
12. Demonstrate evaluation of deep tendon reflexes.
13. Demonstrate evaluation of abnormal reflexes.
14. Differentiate between normal and abnormal speech.
15. Demonstrate evaluation of the ability for abstract thought.
16. Demonstrate evaluation of remote and recent memory.
17. Demonstrate evaluation of mental status.
18. Describe the changes in the nervous system that occur with aging.
19. Describe the variations in the neurological assessment of the infant and child, as compared with the adult.
20. Demonstrate evaluation of pediatric reflexes.
21. Record the findings, using appropriate terminology.

SUGGESTED ACTIVITIES

Read

Alexander, Mary, and Marie Brown: *Pediatric History Taking and Physical Diagnosis for Nurses,* McGraw-Hill, New York, 1979.

Bates, Barbara: "The Neurological System — Adult and Child," *A Guide to Physical Examination,* Lippincott, Philadelphia, 1979.

OR

Malasanos, Lois, et al.: "Neurological Assessment," *Health Assessment,* Mosby, St. Louis, 1977.

Caird, F. I., and T. G. Judge: "Nervous System: History-Taking and Assessment of Mental State," *Assessment of the Elderly Patient,* Pitman, Calif., 1977.

OR

Saxon, Sue V., and Mary Jean Etten: *Physical Change and Aging,* The Tiresias Press, New York, 1978.

View

Bates, Barbara: *Examination of the Neurological System, Parts 1 and 2,* Lippincott videotape, 35 min.

Biological Changes of Aging, Physical Appearance: Special Senses, Trainex (453).

Optional materials

Smith, Kline and French: *Essentials of the Neurological Examination,* Philadelphia, 1968.

Brain model

Equipment

reflex hammer (pediatric size for child)

safety pins (2)

cotton balls

two test tubes (one filled with hot and one filled with cold water)

penlight

tongue depressor

tuning fork

small samples of salt, peanut butter, coffee

coin

cotton-tipped applicator

ticking watch

eye charts

DDST kit, instructions, record form

centimeter tape measure (plastic)

transillumination collar and flashlight (newborn exam only)

ophthalmoscope (for advanced students)

1. The functions of the cerebellar system are to

    a. 1, 3, 4   1. Connect cranial and spinal nerves

    b. 2 and 4 only   2. Receive sensory and motor input

    c. 2, 3, 5   3. Coordinate muscular activity and posture

    d. 1, 2, 5   4. Direct the spinal cord

                            5. Maintain equilibrium

2. Decussation occurs in the _____ _____.

3. The anterior horn cells contain

    a. Sensory neurons

    b. Motor neurons

4. The _____ root contains the sensory fibers.

5. On Fig. 16-1, label the components of the simple reflex arc and the spinal cord sections.

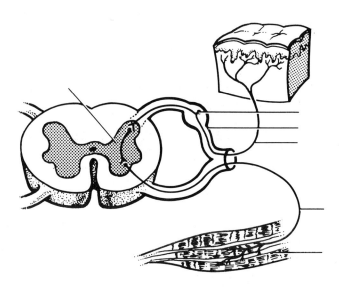

Figure 16-1

6. On Fig. 16-2, label the sections of the brain and the spinal cord, and state the names and numbers of vertebrae in each section.

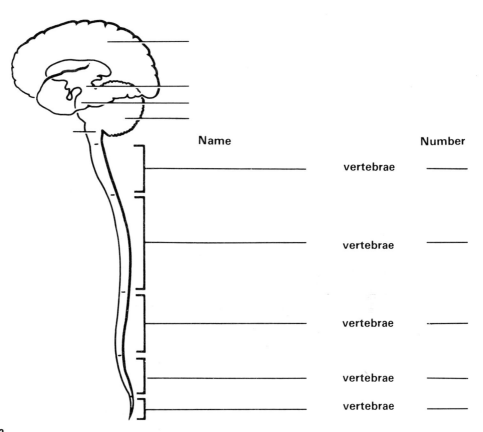

Name   Number

vertebrae ————

vertebrae ————

vertebrae ————

vertebrae ————

vertebrae ————

Figure 16-2

7. Match the following cranial nerve numbers with the appropriate *name* and *function*. (Include all appropriate functions.)

Name	Function	Name	Function
I ____	____	a. Facial	1. Hearing
II ____	____	b. Oculomotor	2. Tongue movement
III ____	____	c. Abducens	3. Sensation in pharynx
IV ____	____	d. Optic	4. Jaw movement
V ____	____	e. Acoustic	5. Vision
VI ____	____	f. Hypoglossal	6. Lateral eye movement
VII ____	____	g. Trigeminal	7. Smell
VIII ____	____	h. Olfactory	8. Downward, medial eye movement
IX ____	____	i. Trochlear	9. Elevation of upper eyelid
X ____	____	j. Vagus	10. Constriction of pupils
XI ____	____	k. Accessory	11. Taste on anterior two-thirds of tongue
XII ____	____	l. Glossopharyngeal	12. Forehead muscle movement
			13. Sternocleidomastoid muscle movement
			14. Posterior tongue sensation, gag reflex
			15. Corneal reflex

8. The segmental level of the triceps deep tendon reflex is _____.

9. Sensations of pain are carried to the brain through the spinothalamic tract on the same side of the spinal column that the stimulation occurred. (True or false? Correct the statement if it is false.)

10. Cerebral functions include which of the following:

a. 1, 2, 4   1. Maintain balance
b. 3, 4, 5   2. Coordinate voluntary movements
c. 2, 3, 4   3. Localization and discrimination among stimuli
d. 2, 4, 5   4. Memory
e. 1, 3, 5   5. Connect cranial and spinal nerves

VOCABULARY   **Descriptive terminology**

agnosia

agraphia

aphasia

apraxia

carphology

clonus

cogwheel rigidity

decerebrate posturing

decorticate posturing

decussation

dysarthria

dysphagia

dysphonia

extinction phenomenon

fasciculation

flaccidity

graphesthesia

kinesthesia

lower motor neuron

nystagmus

paresis (hemiparesis, paraparesis, quadriparesis)

paresthesia

-plegia (monoplegia, hemiplegia, paraplegia, quadriplegia)

point localization

proprioception

spasticity

stereognosis

stereotaxis

tic

tremor

two-point discrimination

upper motor neuron

Diagnostic terminology

Babinski response

Bell's palsy

Brudzinski's sign

chronic brain syndrome

CVA

Kernig's sign

Landau reflex

organic brain syndrome

parkinsonism

Romberg test

DECISION TABLE 16-1

If . . .		Then . . .
You want more information on normal width of sutures and fontanels in infants		*Whole Pediatrician Catalog*, Saunders, Philadelphia, 1977 (newborn chapter).
		Erasmie, V., and H. Ringertz: "Normal Width of Cranial Sutures in the Neonate and Infant," *Acta Radiologics Diagnosis*, **17**:565 ff. (September 5, 1976).
You had difficulty with the cranial nerves		Smith, Kline and French: *Essentials of the Neurological Exam* (pamphlet).
		Test the cranial nerves on several friends, identifying the name, number, and function of each nerve as you test it, until you can do it all without looking at your assessment card.

DECISION TABLE 16-1 (continued)

If . . .		Then . . .

You had difficulty with motor reflexes ⟹ Review Bates.

⟹ Make a chart of the deep tendon reflexes stating how the reflex is elicited, the response, and the segmental level involved.

⟹ DeGowin and DeGowin: *Bedside Diagnostic Examination.*

You had difficulty differentiating cerebellar from cerebral functions ⟹ Review the chapter on brain functions in your anatomy and physiology text.

⟹ Alpers and Mancall: *Essentials of the Neurological Examination,* Davis, Philadelphia, 1971.

You had difficulty with sensory testing ⟹ Alpers and Mancall: *Essentials of the Neurological Examination,* Davis, Philadelphia, 1971.

⟹ Review Bates.

You had difficulty with pediatric adaptations ⟹ Review Bates.

⟹ Review Alexander and Brown.

⟹ Burness, Lewis A.: *Manual of Pediatric Physical Diagnosis,* Year Book, Chicago, 1972.

You seek in-depth coverage of the mental status examination ⟹ Strub, R. L., and F. W. Black: *The Mental Status Examination in Neurology,* Davis, Philadelphia, 1977.

POSTTEST

1. List at least *one* test used to assess the integrity of *each* cranial nerve.

I. _____

II. _____

III. _____

IV. _____

V. _____

VI. _____

VII. _____

VIII. _____

IX. _____

X. _____

XI. _____

XII. _____

2. In the space below, record the following findings using either of the *two* standard recording techniques: "very brisk R biceps and R triceps, diminished L knee and L ankle reflexes, all other reflexes normal." Use tabular form or a stick figure for recording.

3. List the *six* categories of sensation which must be tested.

   a. _____

   b. _____

   c. _____

   d. _____

   e. _____

   f. _____

4. Match the normal response with the appropriate test.

   _____ stepping reflex

   _____ biceps reflex

   _____ plantar reflex

   _____ Moro reflex

   _____ point localization

   _____ Brudzinski's sign

   _____ cremasteric reflex

   _____ knee reflex

   _____ stereognosis

   _____ triceps reflex

   1. Identify two areas of simultaneous stimulation
   2. Contraction of the muscle and elbow extension
   3. Elevation of testicle
   4. Contraction of quadriceps with extension of lower leg
   5. Flexion of toes
   6. Abduction and extension of arms with hands opened then a return to a clasping position
   7. Extension of arms and fingers
   8. Alternate walking movements in response to weight bearing
   9. Contraction of the muscle and flexion of elbow
   10. Identification of area of stimulation
   11. Flexion of hips and knees and pain or resistance on flexion of neck
   12. Identification of an object by feel, not sight

Write *true* or *false*. If *false*, correct the statement to make it true.

5. _____ The rooting reflex is normal in the neonate.

6. _____ Sustained ankle clonus is normal in an infant of any age.

7. _____ Tight closing of the eyes is the response of the glabella reflex in the infant.

8. _____ The Moro reflex is normal in a 10-month-old infant.

9. _____ The brachioradialis reflex causes pronation of the forearm.

10. _____ A deep tendon reflex is not dependent on higher levels of function in the cord and brain.

11. _____ The patellar reflex involves flexion of the knee.

12. _____ An abnormal plantar reflex in an adult would cause dorsiflexion of the great toe and fanning of the other toes.

13. _____ The tendon should be stretched to elicit deep tendon reflex.

14. _____ Abdominal muscle contraction causes the umbilicus to be pulled down in the upper abdominal reflex.

15. _____ The Landau reflex would cause a child to lift the head and extend the spine and legs.

16. _____ Discrimination of hot from cold should be tested only if pain sensation is abnormal.

17. _____ Romberg test is one form of testing cortical function.

18. _____ The deep tendon reflexes of some geriatric clients are delayed or absent.

19. _____ Sensory response to light touch is absent or minimal in geriatric clients.

20. _____ Black children tend to achieve retarded scores for their age on the physical Denver Developmental Screening Test.

21. _____ A history of headaches in a prepubertal child is normal.

22. Which of the following test for general cerebral functioning?
    a. Identification of objects by touch
    b. Perform rapid alternating movements
    c. Perform Romberg test
    d. Differentiate hot from cold temperatures
    e. Demonstrate recall of past, recent, or immediate events

HEALTH HISTORY AND ASSESSMENT

Items marked with an asterisk (*) are to be checked on all clients when doing a complete physical examination; others are to be checked as indicated.

Adult Health History: Neurological System

If the answer is yes, place a check (✔) at the left and provide further information in the Remarks column.

Remarks

_____ Headaches?

_____ Dizziness or fainting?

_____ Loss of consciousness?

_____ Seizures or convulsions?

_____ Numbness, tingling, or decreased sensation?

_____ Twitching muscles?

_____ Muscle weakness or paralysis?

_____ Clumsy or have frequent accidents?

_____ Unsteady? Shaky?

_____ Forgetful? Loss of memory?

_____ Bed-wetting after age 12?

_____ Somnolence?

_____ History of head trauma?

_____ Delayed growth and development?

Adult Physical Assessment— Neurological System

Check (✔) if normal, *NE* if not examined, *X* if abnormal. Describe abnormal findings.

Cranial nerves (see Head and Neck, Modules 4, 5, and 6)

Description

_____ N.I: Correctly identifies odors

_____ *N.II: Normal visual fields

Visual acuity corrected

OD _____ / _____

OS _____ / _____

_____ Optic disks: Within normal limits

_____ *N.III: PERRLA

_____ EOM intact

_____ No ptosis or lid lag

_____ N.IV: Downward medial movement of eyes intact

_____ N.V: Sensory perception of pain, light touch, and temperature are intact in the ophthalmic, maxillary, and mandibular divisions

    _____ Motor function strong with clenched teeth

    _____ Corneal reflexes present

_____ N.VI: Lateral deviation of eye intact

    _____ No nystagmus

_____ *N.VII: Facial muscles strong and symmetrical

    _____ Taste present on anterior tongue

_____ *N.VIII: Auditory acuity normal to ticking watch or whisper

    _____ AC is greater than BC (Rinne)

    _____ No lateralization (Weber)

_____ N.IX, N.X: Normal gag reflex

    _____ Soft palate and uvula symmetrical with upward movement

    _____ Taste present on posterior tongue

_____ N.XI: Sternocleidomastoids and trapezii muscles strong, symmetrical

_____ N.XII: Tongue symmetrical, no deviation, atrophy, or fasciculation

Motor

_____ *Normal gait, heel-to-toe, deep knee bends, walking on heels and toes

_____ *Romberg negative

_____ Good coordination: Finger-to-nose, patting leg, heel-to-shin

_____ Grip strong, no tremor or drift of arms

_____ Muscles — no atrophy, asymmetry, fasciculations, involuntary movements or abnormal positions

_____ Muscles firm, strong: symmetrical strength

Sensory

_____ *Pain perception intact

_____ Perception of light touch, temperature, and vibration intact

_____ Normal position sense and point discrimination

_____ Normal stereognosis and number identification

Mental status and speech

_____ *Orientation to person, place, time

_____ Alert, conscious

_____ Recent and remote memory good

_____ Serial 7s, 3s normal

_____ Able to abstract

_____ Dress and behavior appropriate

_____ Mood _____

Reflexes (0 to 4 scale, normal is 2 +)

_____ *Biceps (C_5, C_6)

_____ *Triceps (C_7, C_8)

_____ *Brachioradialis (C_5, C_6)

_____ Abdominal (T_8, T_9, $T_{10}\uparrow$; T_{10}, T_{11}, $T_{12}\downarrow$)

_____ Cremasteric (L_1, L_2)

_____ *Knee jerk (L_2, L_3, L_4)

_____ *Ankle (S_1, S_2)

_____ Plantar (L_4, L_5, S_1, S_2)

Pediatric Adaptations— History

Paternal history

_____ Age at conception of this child

_____ Blood type

_____ Occupation

_____ Last grade completed in school

_____ Current health problems

_____ Growth patterns of father WNL with respect to age. He

     _____ Walked by 18 months

     _____ Talked by 18 months

     _____ Fed self by 18 months

     _____ Had bowel and bladder control by 3 years

_____ Any paternal history of

     _____ Deafness

     _____ Seizures

     _____ Mental retardation

     _____ Early death of siblings

     _____ Nervous breakdown

     _____ Degenerative illness

     _____ Pregnancy complications of his mother

     _____ Significant illness or surgery

_____ Medications taken prior to conception (hallucinogenic, alcohol, etc.)

Maternal history

_____ Age at conception of this child

_____ Blood type

_____ Occupation

_____ Last grade completed in school

_____ Current health problems

_____ Growth patterns of mother WNL

     _____ Walked by 18 months

     _____ Talked by 18 months

     _____ Fed self by 18 months

     _____ Bowel and bladder control by 3 years

Remarks

_____ Any maternal family history of

     _____ Deafness

     _____ Seizures or convul-
sions

     _____ Mental retardation

     _____ Early death of siblings

     _____ Degenerative illness

     _____ Nervous breakdown

     _____ Pregnancy complica-
tions of her mother

     _____ Previous medical and
surgical events

_____ Good nutrition and diet

_____ Medical supervision

_____ Medications (birth control,
steroids, antibiotics, etc.)

_____

_____ Special treatments or proce-
dures (x-rays, etc.) _____

_____ Complications (bleeding), ill-
nesses or infections (herpes,
VD, measles)

_____ Alcohol consumption

_____ Smoking

_____ X-rays during pregnancy

History of maternal pregnancies

Number	Prenatal care by M.D., R.N., clinic, midwife	Place of birth (hospital home, etc.)	Length of labor	Compli-cations	Route of delivery (vaginal, cesarean section, forceps, pres.)	Sedation, anesthesia required	Birth weights	Problems during first week of life (yellow jaundice, breathing prob-lems, infection, transfusions, etc.)

Prenatal history for this child

_____ Normal delivery

_____ Complications, prematurity

_____ Risk classification

_____ Apgar score (1 min _____
5 min _____)

_____ Birth defects

_____ Bilirubin not over 15 during
first week of life

_____ Childhood illnesses, allergies,
etc.

    _____ Colic

    _____ Feeding problems

    _____ Colds

    _____ Ear trouble

    _____ Wheezing or hoarse-
ness

    _____ Serious falls

    _____ Surgical operations

    _____ Drug reactions

    _____ Skin rashes

    _____ Behavior problems

    _____ Convulsions

    _____ Allergies

_____ Highest fever and duration of
fever

_____ Fever convulsions

_____ Fussy

_____ Tearing of eyes

_____ Easy to manage

_____ Spoiled

_____ Irritable or nervous

_____ Itching

_____ Headaches

_____ Dizziness

_____ Numbness or tingling

_____ Speech problems

_____ Few temper tantrums

_____ Rarely have to spank child

_____ "Overactive"

_____ Stubborn

_____ Likes school

_____ Energetic

_____ Stuttering

_____ Hospitalizations

_____ Immunizations

_____ Broken bones

_____ Accidents or injuries

_____ DPT dates _____

     Reactions _____

_____ Polio dates _____

     Reactions _____

_____ Measles dates _____

     Reactions _____

_____ Rubella dates _____

     Reactions _____

_____ Smallpox dates _____

     Reactions _____

_____ Medications _____

     Reactions _____

_____ Growth patterns and weight changes in months

     _____ Age sat alone

     _____ Age walked alone

     _____ Age talked

     _____ Age fed self

     _____ Age of bowel and bladder control

_____ Speech problems

_____ Sound stimuli in home (radio — volume, etc.)

_____ Good relations between mother and father

_____ Both parents live together

_____ Good father-child relations

_____ Good mother-child relations

_____ Good relations between child and parent substitutes

_____ Good relations with peers

_____ Grade in school (seventh, eighth, etc.)

_____ Generally makes A's, B's, or C's

_____ Adults in home generally agree on the rearing of this child

Diet

_____ Milk type and amount daily

_____ Number of calories daily

_____ Fluid intake daily

_____ Diet includes cereal, milk, vegetables, meat, and fruit

_____ Good appetite

Pediatric Adaptations— Physical

General

Description

_____ Head symmetry

_____ Head circumference in centimeters

_____ Lateral anterior fontanel measurements (up to 16 months)

_____ Vertical anterior fontanel measurements (up to 16 months)

_____ Less than 1 cm transillumination in frontal area of skull; none at occipital base (up to 12 months)

_____ No swelling or nodes palpated on skull

_____ No malformed ears

_____ Ear is on horizontal plane with inner and outer canthus of eye

_____ No cleft lip or palate

Cranial nerves

_____ N.I: Not checked in child under age 2 (have child over age 2 close eyes and identify peanut butter or chocolate)

_____ N.II: Age: Birth
Test: Hold bright object in
front of eyes to attract attention, then move from side to
midline.
Response: Elementary fixation—can follow to the
midline.

_____ Age: 1 to 3 months
Test: Move bright colored
object in front of eyes to attract attention, then move it
through a full 180° range.
Response: Binocular fixa-
tion, follows moving object
through 180°.

_____ Age: 3 to 5 months
Test: Same—also observe
for fixation on distant objects.
Response: Can fixate on objects beyond 3 feet.

_____ Age: 5 to 7 months
Test: Hold the four different
colored Denver Develop-
ment Test blocks in palm
before child.
Response: Prefers red and
yellow.

_____ Age: 7 to 12 months
Test *A*: Attract attention to
raisin held in your palm near
infant.
Test *B*: Begin screening amblyopia by covering each eye
alternately as child observes
raisin or other object.
Response: Fixates on raisin
and will try to pick it up.

_____ Age: 12 to 18 months
Test *A*: Show pictures.
Test *B*: Give pencil and
paper.
Response: Stares at pic-
tures; scribbles on paper.

_____ Age: 18 months to 3 years
Test: Use Denver Eye
Screening Chart.
Response: 20/40 visual
acuity.

_____ Age: 3 to 5 years
Test *A*: Pediatric Eye Chart
or DDST.
Test *B*: Test color discrimination with color blocks.
Test *C*: Test peripheral vision
by having child look straight
ahead as you wiggle your finger in each of the four fields
approaching a 90° angle
from behind.
Response: 20/30 visual
acuity; identifies color by
four years; observes movement at 90° angle.

_____ Age: 6 years
Test: Repeat same process
as above.
Response: 20/20 visual
acuity.

_____ N.III, N.IV: Same as adult.

_____ N.V: Same except blowing
lightly on eyes will elicit corneal reflex in infants and children.
Response: Blinks in response
to blowing on eyes.

_____ N.VI: Nystagmus is normal up
to 4 months.

_____ N.VII: Have child mimic facial
expressions such as frown,
smile, nose wrinkled, eyes
squinting.
Response: Symmetrical movements.

_____ N.VIII: Age: Birth to 4 months
Suspend infant at 30° angle
and rotate each direction in
a complete circle, observing
eye response.
Response: Eyes will oscillate
(nystagmus) in the direction
of rotation.

_____ Age: 4 to 18 months
Test: Attract attention to
silent toy on one side, then
use bell on opposite side
outside of peripheral vi-
sion— orientating-response-
to-noise test. Note response
and repeat on opposite side.
Response: 4 to 5 months—
eyes widen, turns head
slightly in direction of
sound, seems to listen;
6 to 7 months—head turns
toward sound;
8 months—eyes determine
source of sound.

_____ N.IX: Same

_____ N.X: Same

_____ N.XI: Infant—observe head
control.
18 months—have child imitate
shrugging or lifting of
shoulders.

_____ N.XII: Pinch nostrils.
Response: Opens mouth and
raises tip of tongue.

Motor
(For children between ages of 1 month and 5 years give Denver Developmental
Screening Test.)

Observe:

_____ Activity level

_____ Mobility (Walking? Crawling?
Scooting? etc.)

_____ Coordination of spontaneous
and induced movements

_____ Eye-hand coordination

_____ Hand position

_____ Neat pincer grasp (9 months and up)

_____ Good grasp

_____ Resting position

_____ ROM for each major joint to check muscle tone

_____ Coordination while rising from supine to standing position

Sensory

_____ Withdrawal of extremity following painful stimulus

_____ Change in facial expression following painful stimuli

_____ Movement or withdrawal of extremity stimulated by stroking

_____ Vertical suspension positioning

Mental status and speech

_____ Alertness

_____ Quality of cry

Reflexes
(Use semiflexed finger instead of reflex hammer)

_____ Rooting reflex (up to 4 months)

_____ Moro reflex (up to 6 months)

_____ Brudzinski's sign

_____ Kernig's sign

_____ Sucking reflex

_____ Tonic neck reflex (up to 6 months)

_____ Grasp reflex (up to 4 months)

**Geriatric
Adaptations—
Physical**

Description

_____ Startle response delayed

_____ Diminished sense of smell

_____ Diminished sense of taste

_____ Diminished tactile sense

_____ Impaired position sense

_____ Diminished perception of
vibration

_____ Diminished or absent deep
tendon reflexes

_____ Diminished or absent ankle
jerks

_____ Diminished memory for recent
events

_____ Increased time required for responding or reacting to verbal
stimuli

Student_____

INSTRUCTOR'S GUIDE FOR EVALUATION OF STUDENT PERFOR-MANCE

Assessment of the Neurological System

Behaviors evaluated	Yes	No	Remarks
1. Assembles equipment			
2. Takes appropriate history of the neurological system*			
3. Asks branching questions when indicated*			
4. Explains examination procedure to client			
5. Gowns and drapes client to prevent undue exposure			
6. Provides environment free of distractions			
7. Makes notation of client's dress, grooming, personal hygiene, etc.			
8. Checks client's orientation, memory, intellectual performance, judgment, and ability to abstract			
9. Tests olfaction separately for each nostril by occluding the other side			
10. Tests visual acuity correctly			
11. Tests visual fields through six cardinal fields of gaze			
12. Tests extraocular movements and PERRLA			
13. Tests pain and light touch sensation on forehead, cheeks, and jaw on each side of face			
14. Assesses temporal and masseter muscle strength while having client clench teeth			
15. Tests corneal reflex from side, touching *only* the cornea with wisp of cotton			
16. Tests facial symmetry while having client raise eyebrows, frown, smile, show teeth, puff cheeks, and close eyes so they cannot be opened			
17. Tests hearing in each ear separately			
18. Occludes one ear, stands 1 to 2 feet away, covers mouth, and whispers softly or uses ticking watch			
19. Performs Weber's test accurately			
20. Performs Rinne's test accurately			

*If abnormalities are found, a more extensive examination is performed.

Behaviors evaluated	Yes	No	Remarks
21. Assesses gait, including posture, balance, arm swing, steppage			
22. Assesses client's tandem walk			
23. Stands close to client to perform Romberg test, with client's eyes first open, then closed			
24. Assesses client's ability to hop in place, do a shallow knee bend on alternate legs, walk on toes, and walk on heels			
25. Inspects muscles, noting any atrophy, fasciculations, involuntary movements, or abnormalities of position			
26. Tests grip by having client squeeze examiner's crossed index and middle fingers of each hand as hard as possible			
27. Supports client's thigh with one hand while assessing flexion and extension of knee and ankle on each side			
28. Has client close eyes and hold arm straight out in front with palms up for 20 to 30 seconds; notes maintenance of position			
29. Depresses client's outstretched arms alternately against examiner's resistance; notes strength and scapula movement on each side			
30. Has client raise arms over head with palm down and eyes closed for 20 to 30 seconds; notes maintenance of position			
31. Tries to force client's arms down against client's resistance; notes any weakness			
32. Tests flexion and extension of elbow by having client pull and push against examiner's hands			
33. Tests wrist dorsiflexion by having client make a fist and resist examiner's pushing it down			
34. Has client spread fingers and resist examiner trying to force them together			

Behaviors evaluated	Yes	No	Remarks
35. Has client hold thumb tightly against fingertips while examiner pulls own thumb between client's thumb and fingertips; notes strength of client			
36. Observes client during flexion, extension and lateral bending of trunk			
37. Observes excursion of the rib cage and diaphragm during respiration			
38. Tests flexion of hip by placing hand on client's thigh and having client raise leg against it			
39. Tests abduction of hip by placing hands firmly on bed outside client's knees and having client spread legs against examiner's hands			
40. Tests adduction of hip by placing hands firmly on bed between client's knees and having client bring knees together			
41. Tests flexion and extension of knee against resistance			
42. Tests plantar flexion and dorsiflexion at the ankle against resistance			
43. Tests rapid rhythmic alternating movements in each hand and foot			
44. Tests point-to-point movements with hands and legs. Repeats with client's eyes closed			
45. Assesses pain and vibration sense in hands and feet*			
46. Short comparison of light touch with cotton ball over arms and legs*			
47. Uses a familiar small object to test stereognosis with the client's eyes closed*			
48. Checks minimal distance of two-point discrimination			
49. Checks point localization accurately			
50. Checks extinction accurately			
51. Uses reflex hammer accurately			
52. Uses reflex reinforcement techniques appropriately			

*If abnormalities are found, a more extensive examination is performed.

Behaviors evaluated	Yes	No	Remarks
53. Checks following reflexes on each side correctly:			
a. Biceps reflex (C_5, C_6)			
b. Triceps reflex (C_7, C_8)			
c. Brachioradialis (C_5, C_6)			
d. Abdominal reflexes (T_8, T_9, T_{10}, T_{11}, T_{12})			
e. Cremasteric reflexes (L_1, L_2)			
f. Knee reflex (L_2, L_3, L_4)			
g. Ankle reflex (S_1, S_2)			
h. Plantar response (L_4, L_5, S_1, S_2)			
i. Kernig's sign			
j. Brudzinski's sign			
54. Records findings using appropriate terminology			

Instructor _____ Date _____

MODULE 17

PSYCHOLOGICAL ASSESSMENT

Psychological evaluation accompanies and is an integral part of health assessment. Such an evaluation may be made covertly based on verbal and nonverbal data collected during the course of the nurse-client interaction, or it may be made overtly by use of direct questions and systematic use of the mental status examination. Thus, the assessment tools within this module may be completed by carefully analyzing patient behaviors and responses during the history-taking interview and subsequent physical examination, or these assessment tools may be used independently of physical assessment and the client may be directly asked to respond to material presented.

There is a tendency for clients to become defensive and highly anxious if they feel an examiner is questioning and testing mental ability or emotional stability. Therefore, the authors feel that the psychological assessment is *most* effective when the components are integrated throughout the total health assessment. In this fashion, client behaviors and responses can be elicited and observed in the least threatening way. For example, affect, mood, and hygiene can be observed and assessed while interviewing to ascertain the chief complaint or to obtain the social history; mental status can be assessed during the neurological portion of the physical assessment.

As in Module 1, remember that you must focus on patterns in behaviors and responses and must determine what meaning these patterns have for the client. No single behavior alone can tell the story. If speech is slow and halting,

1. Is it because the client speaks another language and must take time to translate responses to English?

2. Is it because the client is elderly and is sorting through vast mental resources to find just the right response?

3. Is it because the client has a neurological deficit; if so, what other behaviors or physical findings are needed for confirmation?

4. Is it because the client has a shortened frenulum and is "tongue-tied"?

5. Is it because the client is having an auditory hallucination and is temporarily distracted by it?

You must continuously practice high-level alertness, and must ask branching questions or make careful observations which seek to validate the meanings behind behaviors observed.

The health history, psychological assessment, and physical examination are best viewed as a whole. Before assumptions can be made about an individual's psychological life, you must know much about the client's psychosocial background and about the physical factors which may impinge upon the individual's well-being. The converse is also true. Therefore, the authors wish to remind you that interpretation of data gathered on the tools within this module will be somewhat limited unless the health history and physical assessment are used in conjunction with and as an adjunct to the psychological evaluation.

Skilled interviewing and observation are necessary for the collection of a psychological assessment. Therefore, you are expected to complete the Pretest in Module 1 before beginning this unit. Otherwise, this module follows the format of the preceding modules.

If you have difficulty or need clarification about the material presented, contact your instructor.

TERMINAL OBJECTIVES

Upon completion of this module you are expected to be able to:

1. Define *life crisis*.
2. Describe the four phases in the development of a crisis.
3. Discuss the relationship between life crisis and the development of anxiety.
4. Contrast situational or accidental crises with maturational or developmental crises.
5. Define *anxiety*.
6. Describe the development of anxiety as it leads to personality disorganization.
7. Identify defense mechanisms used to cope with anxiety.
8. Describe behaviors representing a psychological response to anxiety.
9. Describe physiological responses to anxiety.
10. Identify the major elements of a psychological assessment.
11. Identify components of the assessment of general behavior and appearance.
12. Identify components of the assessment of the sensorium.
13. Identify components of the assessment of cognitive skills.
14. Describe methods of assessing emotional status and affect.

15. Describe the use of "self-drawings" in assessment of body image.
16. Discuss the relationship between the psychological portion of the data-gathering interview and the remainder of the health history and physical assessment.
17. Given an assessment form, conduct a psychological assessment.
18. Record findings using appropriate terminology.
19. Utilizing the data collected, identify patterns in the behavior of a client.

SUGGESTED ACTIVITIES

Read

The chapters on anxiety, defense mechanisms, life crises, neurosis, psychoses, and depression in a psychiatric nursing textbook.

OR

Grace, Helen K., et al.: *Mental Health Nursing: A Sociopsychological Approach,* Wm. C. Brown Company Publishers, Dubuque, Iowa, 1977, pp. 53-78, 87-107, 158-163, 202-209.

OR

Mereness, Dorothy, and Cecilia Monat Taylor: *Essentials of Psychiatric Nursing,* Mosby, St. Louis, 1978, pp. 29-73, 147-163, 182-213, 215-225, 227-239, 240-277.

AND

Bates, Barbara: "Mental Status," *A Guide to Physical Examination,* Lippincott, Philadelphia, 1979.

OR

Malasanos, Lois, et al.: "Neurological Assessment: Mental Status," *Health Assessment,* Mosby, St. Louis, 1977.

View

Psychological Defenses, Series A — Unconscious, Harper & Row filmstrip with sound (IFS 40A).

Psychological Defenses, Series A — Avoidance, et al., Harper & Row filmstrip with sound (IFS 40B).

Psychological Defenses, Series A — Fantasy, et al., Harper & Row filmstrip with sound (IFS 40C).

Psychological Defenses, Series B — Projection, et al., Harper & Row filmstrip with sound (IFS 40D).

Psychological Defense, Series B — Identification, et al., Harper & Row filmstrip with sound (IFS 40E).

Psychological Defenses, Series B — Reaction Formation, et al., Harper & Row filmstrip with sound (IFS 40F).

Psychosocial Assessment, Part 2, American Journal of Nursing Co. video cassette. (This videotape shows an actual interview in progress. It provides an opportunity to identify major themes and psychological responses of a client in an interview situation.)

Equipment

psychiatric glossary or dictionary

VOCABULARY   **Descriptive terminology**

affect	euphoria
flattened	facies
inappropriate	"flight of ideas"
agraphia	grief
alexia	hallucination
ambivalence	hysteria
amnesia	identification
anomia	illusion
anxiety	insight
aphasia	intellectualize
autism	introjection
circumlocution	judgment
clang association	mental dysfunction
compensation	obsession
compulsion	oriented
cognitive skills	panic
confabulation	paranoia
confusion	phobia
conversion reaction	projection
coping style	rationalization
crisis	reaction formation
accidental or situational	reality testing
developmental or maturational	repression
delirium	sensorium
delusions	somnolent
of persecution	somatization
of reference	subject-object differentiation
of grandeur	sublimation
denial	suicidal
depersonalization	suppression
disorientation	thought
displacement	circumstantial
dissociative reaction	perseverated
dysarthria	incoherent
dyslexia	primary process
dysphonia	undoing
dysphagia	waxy flexibility
dysprosody	word salad
ego boundaries	
ESP	

Descriptive terminology

anxiety reaction	mental retardation	psychoses	sociopathic
depression	neuroses	psychotic	
manic-depressive	paranoid	schizophrenic	

DECISION TABLE 17-1

If . . .		Then . . .
You wish further information on the role of anxiety in influencing mental status	⟹	"Anxiety: Recognition and Intervention," *American Journal of Nursing,* **65**:130(1965) (programmed instruction).
	⟹	Peplau, Hildegard E.: "A Working Definition of Anxiety," *Some Clinical Approaches to Psychiatric Nursing,* S. F. Burd and M. A. Marshall (eds.), Macmillan, New York, 1963, pp. 323-327.
You wish further assistance with mental defense mechanisms and enjoy programmed instruction	⟹	"Understanding Defense Mechanisms," *American Journal of Nursing,* 1651-1674 (September, 1972).
You would like three general overviews of the mental status or psychiatric examination	⟹	Stevenson, Ian: "The Psychiatric Interview" and "The Psychiatric Examination," *American Handbook of Psychiatry,* S. Arieta (ed.), Basic Books, New York, 1967, pp. 197-237.
	⟹	Bell, Richard, and Richard Hall: "The Mental Status Examination," *American Family Physician,* **16**:145-152 (November, 1977).
	⟹	Prior, John A., and Jack S. Silberstein: *Physical Diagnosis,* Mosby, St. Louis, 1977, pp. 36-53.
You wish a brief look at the key elements in a psychological assessment	⟹	Snyder, Joyce C., and Margaret Wilson: "Elements of a Psychological Assessment," *American Journal of Nursing,* 236-239 (February, 1977).
You are fascinated and want an in-depth, detailed discussion of the components of the psychological assessment	⟹	Francis, Gloria, and Barbara A. Munjas: *Manual of Social-Psychologic Assessment,* Appleton-Century-Crofts, New York, 1976, pp. 105-173.
You need to understand the effect of territoriality on behavior	⟹	Stillman, Margot J.: "Territoriality and Personal Space," *American Journal of Nursing,* 1670-1672 (October, 1978).
You wish an excellent reference and are a more advanced student	⟹	Strub, Richard L., and F. William Black: *The Mental Status Examination in Neurology,* Davis, Philadelphia, 1977.
You are seeking a general discussion of emotional disorders of childhood and adolescence	⟹	Clements, C. Glenn: "Emotional disorders of Childhood and Adolescence With Some Implications for Nursing," *Basic Psychiatric Concepts in Nursing,"* Joan Kyes and Charles Hofling (eds.), Lippincott, Philadelphia, 1974, pp. 360-393.

DECISION TABLE 17-1 (continued)

If . . .		Then . . .
You wish a discussion of psychological disturbances in the aged	⟹	Burnside, Irene: "Mental Health in the Aged," "Acute and Chronic Brain Syndromes," "Depression and Suicide in the Aged," *Nursing and the Aged,* I. Burnside (ed.), McGraw-Hill, New York, 1976, pp. 136–181.
	⟹	Burnside, Irene Mortenson: "Recognizing and Reducing Emotional Problems in the Aged," *Nursing '77,* 56–59 (March, 1977).
	⟹	Butler, Robert, and Myrna Lewis: *Aging and Mental Health,* Mosby, St. Louis, 1977, pp. 34–91.
	⟹	Caird, F. I., and T. G. Judge: *Assessment of the Elderly Patient,* Pitman, Calif., 1977, pp. 87–98.
You wish to evaluate the mental status of a confused patient	⟹	Dodd, Marylin J.: "The Confused Patient: Assessing Mental Status," *American Journal of Nursing,* 1501–1503 (September, 1978).
You are working in an intensive-care unit and wish to conduct a mental status exam; see how this one is designed	⟹	Adams, Margaret, et al.: "The Confused Patient: Psychological Responses in Critical Care Units," *American Journal of Nursing,* 1504–1512 (September, 1978).
You are an advanced student and wish a source which will help in the assessment and management of psychosocial problems and emotional disturbances	⟹	Capell, Peter, and David B. Case: *Ambulatory Care for Nurse Practitioners,* Lippincott, Philadelphia, 1976, pp. 237–258.

POSTTEST

Write *true* or *false.* If *false,* correct the statement to make it true.

1. _____ Crises force individuals to develop a change in their coping styles.

2. _____ A crisis occurs when an individual can no longer use usual problem-solving patterns to resolve a problem and is unable to invoke a more productive pattern.

3. _____ Crises may be divided into two major categories—situational and accidental.

4. _____ Depression is related to a loss of something the individual values and is a manifestation of the grief over that loss.

5. _____ Delusions and hallucinations develop through the process of introjection.

6. _____ Words strung together because of how they sound and not what they mean are termed *word salad.*

7. _____ In performing the psychological assessment, the examiner is seeking to observe patterns in behavior.

8. _____ Recent memory may be assessed by having client repeat five to eight digits forward and four to six digits backward.

9. _____ Asking the client to relate the meaning of familiar proverbs is a method of assessing affect.

10. _____ Disturbance in the understanding or expression of words is termed *dyslexia.*

Match the descriptions in the right column with the terms in the left column.

11. _____ Repression

12. _____ Phobia

13. _____ Hallucination

14. _____ Reaction formation

15. _____ Autism

16. _____ Projection

17. _____ Ambivalence

18. _____ Introjection

19. _____ Compulsion

20. _____ Denial

21. _____ Anxiety reaction

22. _____ Depersonalization

a. A false sensory perception without an apparent basis in reality

b. Refusal to admit the existence of unpleasant reality

c. Simultaneous presence of opposite feelings toward some person or goal

d. Warding off anxiety by adopting certain attitudes and behaviors of other people

e. Automatic forgetting that occurs at times of severe anxiety

f. Uncontrollable, persistant desire to perform a certain behavior

g. Sense of impending doom

h. Subjective experience of being isolated or removed from the reality surrounding oneself

i. Wishes or feelings associated with initial anxiety that are transformed to their opposites

j. Unacceptable wishes or feelings that are assigned to someone else

k. Persistent fear of a specific place or thing which is impossible to banish from the mind

l. Extreme preoccupation with the self and an accompanying withdrawal from external connections or interests, including people

23. List *four* physical manifestations of anxiety.

a. _____

b. _____

c. _____

d. _____

24. Categorize the following descriptions of behavior as examples of *mild, moderate,* or *severe* anxiety.

   a. Client cannot make connections between details or see the "whole picture" formed by such a connection (cannot see the forest for the trees). _____

   b. Client distorts and enlarges details and cannot communicate thoughts and feelings to the examiner in a way that they can be understood. _____

   c. Client is well oriented to reality and exhibits an awareness of events transpiring in the environment; client can observe and verbalize insights concerning own behavior. _____

   d. Client concentrates on relevant details within a limited sphere of awareness, but may selectively disregard much of what is transpiring in the environment. _____

25. Listed below are 15 client behaviors observed by an examiner. Note whether the behavior would be considered normal (*N*) or would require further evaluation and possible referral (*R*).

   a. _____ The client, a physician's wife, appears for the interview in the nurse's outpatient office wearing soiled and torn clothing and with an unkempt appearance (dirty stringy hair, dirty nails, and no makeup).

   b. _____ When the nurse offers a cup of coffee, the client refuses, exclaiming, "No! My family is trying to poison me and you are in with them."

   c. _____ During the interview the client sits, seldom responding, with head tilted as though listening to something far away. The client seems to be in another world.

   d. _____ During a fairly lengthy description of his wife's long illness and subsequent death, Mr. Smith smiles and occasionally breaks into periods of overt laughter.

   e. _____ A 4-year-old child tells you what an imaginary playmate looks like and about their adventures the preceding day.

   f. _____ A 55-year-old client relates to you the events that ended her 25-year marriage, which included her husband's abrupt departure with his 22-year-old secretary. You note that her face shows little or no expression and that her fists remain clenched during this recital. However, she further describes her husband as wonderful, fine, loving, and concerned only with her well-being.

   g. _____ A student, who has recently been suspended from college due to poor grades, describes herself as unable to sleep at night, except intermittently, and unable to get going during the day. She states she has no energy and cares little about her surroundings or activities.

h. _____ Mr. Smith, a 79-year-old retired railroad worker brought to the outpatient clinic, responds to the nurse's question, "Do you know where you are, Mr. Smith?" with the answer, "Why, of course. I'm at the Penn Central Station. Got to get the mail ready for the night train; it's coming through in an hour."

i. _____ Mrs. Elliot, aged 81, frequently responds appropriately to questions asked by the examiner, but also likes to interrupt the interview and tell little stories about her past.

j. _____ Mrs. Spock reports that she is concerned about her daughter Julie, aged 6, who seems to derive pleasure from pulling the dog's tail, lifting it by the ears, and twisting its legs.

k. _____ Ryan, aged 2, is brought to the nurse, who is told by the boy's mother, "I don't know what is wrong with Ryan. He keeps having 'accidents' [wets his pants]."

l. _____ Mrs. Little, aged 86, is brought to the nurse by her daughter who complains, "Mother is losing her mind — she can remember everything that happened in 1900, but can't remember where she went yesterday or where she hung her coat this morning."

m. _____ Miss Francis, aged 81, is bright and alert, and relates delightful stories to the nurse concerning her days as a small-town librarian. She complains that she has noticed a change in her patterns of sleep in the last few years. She finds that she is awake much of the night and sleeps only 5 or 6 hours — she does admit to an occasional nap during the day.

n. _____ Jack Whittier, aged 25, a college graduate, responding to the examiner's request to explain "a stitch in time saves nine," answers, "It takes less thread to make one stitch than nine."

o. _____ When asked to draw a picture of himself, 12-year-old Burt completes this picture and gives it to the nurse.

Indicate what facets of psychological integrity the examiner is evaluating by requesting the following client responses or by noting the following client behaviors:

26. _____ The examiner asks the client to repeat the following digits in reverse order: 4, 9, 3, 2, 8, 7, 1.

27. _____ The examiner observes that a client misidentifies a teddy bear as being her baby.

28. _____ The examiner instructs the client to begin at 100, subtract 7, and keep subtracting 7.

29. _____ The examiner asks for the client's own name and the names of close relatives.

30. _____ The client is asked to copy geometric figures drawn by the examiner.

31. _____ The examiner asks the client, "If you bought six candy bars at 20 cents each and gave the grocer a $5 bill, how much change would you expect?"

32. _____ The examiner asks the client, "Do you ever feel that people are out to get you?"

33. _____ The examiner observes that the client consistently cannot follow instructions during the physical examination.

34. _____ The examiner asks an adult, "What did you have for breakfast today?"

35. _____ The examiner asks the client, "What would you do if you were stopped for speeding?"

36. _____ The examiner observes that the client's facial expression remains waxy and immobile during the interview—no changes in features or expression are noted.

37. _____ The examiner asks the client to tell the examiner how a hoe and a wrench are alike.

38. _____ The examiner asks the client, "Have you ever thought of doing away with yourself?"

39. _____ The examiner asks an adult client, "Tell me about your childhood."

40. _____ The examiner observes that a male client is dressed, shaved, and groomed impeccably on the left side, but the right side of his face is unshaven, his shirt cuff is unbuttoned, and his right shoe and sock are missing.

41. _____ The examiner notes that as a client responds to questions, she becomes lost in reporting minute details and forgets the questions asked by the examiner.

42. _____ The examiner rings a small bell and asks the client to identify the sound made.

43. _____ The examiner asks the client, "What day of the week is this? What month of the year? What time of day?"

44. _____ The examiner notes that the client's speech is slurred and halting.

45. _____ The examiner presents nine digits, 7, 3, 9, 8, 2, 1, 6, 5, 4, and asks the client to repeat them in the order presented.

46. _____ The examiner observes that while the client is describing the funeral of his child and the tragedy that led to this event, he smiles and laughs.

47. _____ The examiner observes that the client's face is flushed, client's palms are clammy and cold, and client constantly twists handkerchief during interview.

48. _____ The examiner asks the client, "Can you tell me where you are now? What town you live in? What state?"

49. _____ The examiner asks the client to tell the examiner the meaning of the following: "A bird in the hand is worth two in the bush."

50. _____ The examiner observes that the client seems extremely withdrawn, responds to questions slowly — if at all — does not make eye contact, and states that she feels sad.

HEALTH HISTORY AND ASSESSMENT

If the answer is yes, place a check (✓) at the left and provide further information in the Remarks column.

Psychological History

Remarks

Do you

_____ Walk in your sleep?

_____ Experience dreamlike periods when you do things you do not remember?

_____ Sometimes feel that you are another person doing things?

_____ Write things automatically?

_____ Find you cannot concentrate or pay attention to anything for very long?

_____ Forget what you were going to say in the middle of a sentence?

_____ Find yourself dwelling on something so much that it interferes with other activities?

_____ Have episodes of ESP (extrasensory perception)?

_____ See or hear things that others say are not there?

_____ Others say you experience things differently from the way they are?

_____ Smell, taste, or feel things that you or others believe are imaginary?

_____ Feel that your body is displeasing?

_____ Have periods of feeling separated from everything else?

_____ Feel that you are watching yourself?

_____ Feel that things are happening around you with no meaning?

_____ Feel unreal or that things around you are unreal?

_____ Have trouble controlling your anger?

_____ Have frequent blue spells?

_____ Have bouts of depression?

_____ Experience frequent changes of mood?

_____ Tend to get high and excited?

_____ Ever feel like giving up?

_____ Have thoughts of killing yourself?

_____ Term yourself nervous or anxious?

_____ Get your feelings hurt easily?

_____ Feel apathetic, detached, indifferent?

_____ Often feel lonely?

_____ Feel you can't communicate with others?

_____ Have trouble getting to the point in conversation?

_____ Feel awkward in social situations?

_____ Find yourself seeking solitude much of the time?

_____ Spend so much time daydreaming that it interferes with your life?

_____ Have thoughts that others laugh at?

_____ Have thoughts that run through your mind that you can't get out?

_____ Have fears that bother you?

_____ Have trouble remembering things that happened recently?

_____ Remember things from long ago better than recent events?

_____ Have a specific event for which you have no memory?

_____ Often feel that something you are experiencing has happened before?

_____ Hear voices that are not there?

_____ Feel you are being manipulated by others?

_____ Often feel that others don't like you?

_____ Often feel that others are talking about you?

_____ Term yourself _a leader_?

_____ Term yourself _a follower_?

_____ Feel overly involved in religious or spiritual affairs?

_____ Have difficulty making decisions?

_____ Have a history of head injury?

_____ Have a history of neurological disease?

_____ Have a history of problems with your nerves?

_____ Have problems with your physical health that seem to be caused or aggravated by stress (example: ulcer, hives, diarrhea)?

_____ Take medication? If so, what?

_____

_____

_____ Use mind-altering drugs or experiences?

_____ Have frequent experiences of light-headedness?

_____ Experience blackouts?

_____ Have a history of:

_____ Headaches?

_____ Coma?

_____ Neurological or brain surgery?

_____ Cerebrovascular accident (stroke)?

_____ Episodes of prolonged high fever?

_____ Convulsions or epilepsy?

_____ ECT/EST treatments?

_____ Receiving psychotherapy?

_____ Neurological or psychological disease in your family?

_____ Diabetes or other metabolic disorder?

_____ Developmental delays or problems (example: delayed walking, talking, school problems)?

_____ Aggressive or violent behavior?

_____ Arrests or treatment for sexual deviation, antisocial behavior, violence?

_____ Have periods of physical or mental exhaustion?

_____ Drink alcoholic beverages?

Has there been any recent change in

_____ Your activity level?

_____ Sleeping habits?

_____ Eating habits?

_____ Bowel habits?

_____ Sexual activity?

_____ Mood?

_____ Relationships with family members?

_____ Relationships with coworkers?

_____ Relationships with friends?

_____ Ability to perform functions required by job or school?

_____ Ability to read or perform mathematical calculations?

Other comments or remarks you would like to make:

Pediatric Adaptations— History

Remarks

_____ Results of Denver Developmental Screening Test (DDST) within normal limits for age?

_____ Results of Pre-School Readiness Experimental Screening Scale (PRESS) within normal limits?

_____ No developmental delays?

_____ No history of brain damage at birth?

_____ No history of prolonged labor at birth?

_____ No history of prematurity?

_____ No history of Rh incompatibility at birth?

_____ No history of rubella, syphilis, etc., of mother during pregnancy?

_____ No history of asthma, hives, rhinitis, or other allergic responses?

_____ No history of gastric distrubances, colitis, vomiting, anorexia, stomachaches?

_____ No history of failure to thrive?

_____ No history of headaches, head trauma?

_____ Parent reports no recent changes in behavior?

_____ Child establishes eye contact with parent?

_____ Child establishes eye contact with examiner?

_____ Attention span within normal limits for age?

_____ Infant: Responds to familiar objects (mother's face, bottle)?

_____ Recalls digits presented by examiner?

      Age 4: Recalls 3

      Age 5: Recalls 4

      Age 6: Recalls 5

_____ Recent memory intact (can name object presented by examiner 5 min before)?

_____ Remote memory intact: Can recall birthday, what had for dinner last night?

_____ No feeding difficulties?

_____ Not taking bottle beyond age 3?

_____ No daytime toilet accidents in clothes beyond age 3?

_____ No enuresis beyond age 4?

_____ No disturbances in bowel patterns or habits (holding, fecal smearing)?

_____ No disturbances in sleep patterns or habits?

_____ No somnambulism?

_____ No phobias?

_____ Relates to age of others appropriately?

_____ Has and interacts with playmates own age?

_____ No problems reported with siblings?

_____ No problems reported between parents and child?

_____ Speech present and appropriate for age?

_____ No abnormal speech patterns (example: stuttering or stammering)?

_____ No history of reading difficulties?

_____ No history of functioning below level of intelligence?

_____ No history of truancy?

_____ Flexible and responds appropriately to change?

_____ Does not regress to behaviors of earlier age when confronted with problems?

_____ No history of hyperactivity?

_____ Infrequent injuries and accidents?

_____ No self-destructive behavior?

_____ No history of destructiveness to property?

_____ Not cruel to people or animals?

_____ No history of discipline problems?

No excessive

- _____ Violence or aggression
- _____ Withdrawal
- _____ Daydreaming
- _____ Staring
- _____ Head-banging
- _____ Rocking
- _____ Thumb-sucking
- _____ Encopresis
- _____ Nail-biting
- _____ Teeth-grinding
- _____ Attachment to imaginary playmates
- _____ Attachment to inanimate objects
- _____ Self-manipulation of body/sexual organs
- _____ Tics
- _____ Involvement with inappropriate playmates
- _____ Fantasy life
- _____ Drowsiness or lethargy
- _____ Temper tantrums

Describe quality of interaction between parent and child during the interview:

Geriatric Adaptations— History

Remarks

_____ Loss of memory for recent events, or acute recall of events of early life?

_____ Tendency to reminisce?

_____ Failure to respond readily to change?

_____ Alteration of sleep-wakeful- ness patterns (naps during day; is more sleepless at night than had been in younger years)?

Psychological Assessment: Mental Status

General description of client (include in overview a _brief_ description of facies, posture, general behavior, grooming and apparel, handedness—right, left, or am- bidextrous):

Attitude of client toward interviewer (give behavioral example to support comment):

Check (✔) if normal, _NE_ if not examined, _X_ if abnormal. Describe all abnormal find- ings. Support all conclusions with examples of client behavior.

Mood or affect

Description

_____ No inappropriate or flattened affect

Based on personal observation and interaction, how would you describe the client's pres- ent mood?

_____

Appearance and general behavior

_____ Body movements coordinated; no unusual postures or mannerisms

_____ Hygiene good

_____ Clothing appropriate for time and place

_____ Cosmetics applied appropriately

_____ No inappropriate territorial distancing

_____ No disturbance in motor activity

_____ No impairment in fine motor coordination (can copy geometric figures)

_____ Able to maintain eye contact

_____ No unusual eye or pupillary movements

_____ Facial expression mobile

_____ Voice well modulated — pitch intensity controlled

_____ Inflection of voice varies and is related to ideas being expressed

_____ Word flow smooth and moderately paced

_____ Operates with mutuality during interaction (no monopolizing or withdrawal from interaction)

Sensorium

_____ Oriented to time, place, person

_____ Alert and attentive

_____ Responds appropriately to questions

_____ Able to repeat five to eight digits forward; four to six backward

_____ No impairment of remote memory

_____ No disturbance in clarity of consciousness

_____ Awareness of inner life experiences intact (is able to recognize and describe own feelings)

_____ Subject-object differentiation intact (does not confuse objects with each other or confuse objects with persons)

_____ Ego boundaries intact

_____ Recognizes, differentiates, and associates external stimuli

_____ Perceives visual stimuli accurately (copies written word)

_____ Perceives auditory stimuli (can accurately identify sounds presented by examiner)

_____ Perceives tactile stimuli accurately (identifies objects presented by examiner)

_____ Responds to visual, auditory, tactile stimuli bilaterally (no failure to pay attention to stimuli on one side of body — unilateral neglect)

_____ No preoccupation or distortion of thought

_____ Thinking moves in steady progression toward goal

_____ Able to adapt to new situations

_____ Displays awareness of present situation

Cognitive skills

_____ Ability to abstract is present (when presented with four proverbs is able to abstractly interpret at least two)

_____ Comprehension is present

_____ Able to determine similarities

_____ Demonstrates ability to learn or read

_____ Computational ability intact (demonstrates by serial 7s or 3s)

_____ Displays wide range of information

_____ Utilizes vocabulary appropriately in expressing self

_____ Demonstrates ability to solve problems; exercises judgment in decision making

_____ Exhibits ability to cooperate in preventive care or treatment program

Predominant themes or patterns of behavior of client noted during interaction:

Areas consistently avoided or blocked during interaction:

Predominant nonverbal behaviors:
  Mannerisms (nail-biting, smoking, etc.):
  Physiological changes (flushing, perspiring, etc.):

Body image as exhibited by self-drawing:

Client's view or description of his or her own life at present:

Future goals or plans of client:

Support the following evaluations with a behavioral example:

Anxiety level during interaction: Low _____ Medium _____ High _____

Self-esteem of client: High _____ Average _____ Low _____

Intelligence level of client: High _____ Average _____ Low _____ Retarded _____

Present growth and developmental level of client:

Results of psychological tests:

Recommendations, treatment, or disposition of abnormal findings:

Student _____

INSTRUCTOR'S GUIDE FOR EVALUATION OF STUDENT PERFOR-MANCE

Psychological Assessment

Note to instructor: Abnormal behavior is unlikely to be exhibited when the student interviews another student in the laboratory to obtain a psychological assessment. Therefore, one of the following approaches is suggested in evaluating student performance:

1. *Role play.* Two faculty members will be required in the use of this approach. One will serve as the evaluator of the student-client interaction. The second will serve as the client who will exhibit normal and abnormal behavior during a 10-min nurse-client interview. Prior to the role playing, specific behavioral actions may be decided upon by the faculty and rehearsed and perfected to convey these behaviors to the student. The student will be evaluated on identification and description of behaviors occurring during the interaction.

2. *Videotape of nurse-client interaction.* A videotape may be made of a nurse conducting a simulated mental status examination. The student would be expected to complete the psychological assessment form based on behaviors and abilities exhibited by the client in the course of the interview. Such a tape should run no longer than 30 min, and the assessment could be completed prior to the scheduled final evaluation date. Laboratory time could be used by the faculty member to review results of the assessment.

If the psychological assessment is conducted in conjunction with the health assessment interview, both components of the assessment should be considered as one in the evaluation. The setting and ostensible purpose for the nurse-patient interaction should be the history-taking interview since the psychological assessment is most often completed at this time.

Behaviors evaluated	Yes	No	Remarks
1. Introduces self to client and explains the the purpose of the interview			
2. Provides an environment conducive to effective interviewing (comfortable, quiet, etc.)			
3. Treats client with respect and concern			
4. Maintains focus of interview on client and client's concerns			
5. Uses facilitative interviewing techniques (open-ended questions, clarification and redirection of conversation when it strays, transitional statements, etc.)			
6. Identifies themes in client conversation			

Behaviors evaluated	Yes	No	Remarks
7. Identifies inappropriate responses to questions and disorders in thought displayed in answers			
8. Identifies impairment in memory			
9. Assesses cognitive skills (if indicated, may use serial 7s and 3s, vocabulary test, assessment of range of general information, and ability to abstract)			
10. Evaluates sensory perception and fine motor coordination			
11. Identifies discrepancies in verbal and nonverbal behavior			
12. Identifies inappropriate behaviors or mannerisms exhibited in the interview situation			
13. Assesses body image of client			
14. Evaluates anxiety level of client			
15. If client questionnaire is used, reviews results with client			
16. Evaluates the impact of own behavior in the nurse-client interview			

Instructor _____ Date _____

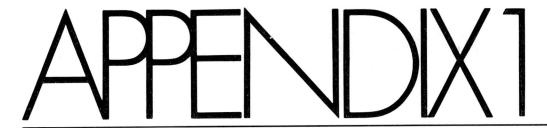

MODEL ADULT HEALTH HISTORY FORM

Client _____ Date _____

Sex: M _____ F _____ Birth date _____ Age _____

Race _____ Language spoken _____

Chief complaint

History of present illness

Onset _____

Precipitating factor _____

Potentiating factor _____

Relieving factor _____

Past treatment or evaluation of symptom _____

Location/duration _____

Quality/quantity _____

Course of the symptom _____

Effect on normal daily activities_____

Other _____

Past history

Serious illnesses _____

Surgeries _____

Trauma _____

Infectious diseases: mumps, rubella, rubeola, chickenpox, pertussis, influenza,
    tuberculosis, mononucleosis, venereal disease, common cold, other_____

_____

Other illnesses: Arthritis, seizures, pneumonia, diabetes, thyroid disease, heart
    disease, hypertension, renal disease, liver disease, ulcer, colitis, anemia, cancer or
    tumor, other _____

Immunizations (date):

    diphtheria and tetanus _____   influenza _____

    polio _____   smallpox _____

    rubella _____   tine or PPD _____

    rubeola _____   other_____

    mumps _____

Allergies, food and drug reactions _____

Blood transfusions _____

Foreign travel _____

Current medications _____

Family history

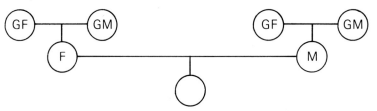

Identify familial history of: Diabetes mellitus, tuberculosis, cancer, stroke, hyper-
    tension, heart disease, vascular disease, anemia, renal disease, emphysema, liver
    disease, ulcers, glaucoma, deafness, gout, arthritis, allergies, birth defects,
    epilepsy, mental retardation, mental health problems, alcoholism, accident
    proneness, obstetric difficulties

Legend: ● *Cause* = deceased   ○ *L&W* = living and well

                                           ○ *Disease* = living, with disease listed

Review of Systems

If the answer is *yes,* place a check (✔) at the left and provide further information in the Remarks column.

General overview   Remarks

General health _____

_____

_____ Have you lost or gained weight? How much?

_____ Chronically tired?

_____ Difficulty going to sleep or staying asleep?

_____ Chills, fever, aching?

_____ Frequently too hot? Too cold?

Skin

_____ Recent change in warts or moles?

_____ Any skin diseases?

_____ Subject to athlete's foot?

_____ Any swelling, lump, or sore on body?

_____ Rashes?

_____ Itching?

_____ Skin dry?

_____ Excessive sweating?

_____ Any change in temperature of skin?

_____ Any unusual discoloration or pigmentation of skin?

_____ Change in pigmentation or color?

_____ Easy bleeding or bruising?

_____ Delayed healing of wounds?

_____ Easy to sunburn?

_____ Any tenderness or pain?

_____ Recent loss of hair?

_____ Any change in hair growth or texture?

_____ Problem with dandruff or scaling?

_____ Any color changes in nails?

Head and neck

_____ Severe headaches or head pains?

_____ Dizziness or fainting?

_____ Head injury?

_____ Pain or stiffness in neck?

_____ Swelling or enlarged glands?

_____ Goiter or thyroid trouble?

_____ Need to take thyroid medicine?

Eyes

_____ Any disturbance in vision?

_____ Wear glasses?

_____ Pain, burning, itching?

_____ Redness or discharge?

_____ Eye problems (glaucoma, cataract, stye, infection)?

Ears

_____ Hard of hearing?

_____ Constant noise in ears?

_____ Chronic running ear?

_____ Earaches with colds or plane flights?

_____ Stopped-up?

_____ Chronic itching?

Nose and sinuses

_____ Chronic stuffy or runny nose?

_____ Loss of smell?

_____ Chronic drip from nose to throat?

_____ Frequently use nose drops?

_____ Nosebleeds?

Mouth and throat

_____ Frequent colds or sore throat?

_____ Need to clear throat frequently?

_____ Hoarseness at times?

_____ Any known dental problems?

_____ More than a year since teeth checked?

_____ Sore mouth or tongue?

Gastrointestinal

_____ Poor appetite?

_____ Nausea or vomiting?

_____ Vomiting of blood?

_____ Indigestion, heartburn, or food intolerance?

_____ Belching, gas?

_____ Yellow skin or eyes?

_____ Burning or hunger pains in stomach?

_____ Difficulty in swallowing?

_____ Soreness, pain, or cramps in abdomen?

_____ Diarrhea?

_____ Constipation?

_____ Black or tarry stools?

_____ Mucus in stools?

_____ Use laxatives or enemas frequently?

_____ Recent change in bowel habits?

_____ Rectal trouble or pain?

_____ Family history of colitis, ulcers, or enteritis?

Drugs taken_____

Foods that disagree _____

Cardiovascular and pulmonary

_____ Worried about your heart?

_____ Ever told that your blood pressure was too high? _____

Too low? _____

_____ Pain in heart or chest?

_____ Heart pounding or skipping a beat?

_____ Heart starts racing suddenly?

_____ Ever told you had a murmur?

_____ Any shortness of breath?

_____ Require more than one pillow for sleeping?

_____ Sudden shortness of breath at night?

_____ Coughing up sputum?

_____ Ever coughed up blood-tinged sputum?

_____ Recent or chronic cough?

_____ Shortness of breath or wheezing?

_____ Difficulty in breathing?

_____ Ever have to sit up to breathe?

_____ Urination during the night? How many times? _____

_____ Swelling of ankles or hands?

_____ Dizziness or fainting?

_____ Numbness or tingling of arms or legs?

_____ Leg cramps in bed or sitting still?

_____ Leg cramps while walking?

_____ Chills or fever?

_____ Night sweats?

_____ Long-term exposure to industrial dust, coal dust, asbestos?

_____ Do you smoke? Number per day? _____

_____ Taking medicine for heart or blood pressure? What?_____

_____ Previous ECG? Date_____

_____ Chest x-ray? Date _____

Breasts and axillae

_____ Enlargement, tenderness, or lumps?

_____ Nipple discharge?

_____ Monthly breast examination?

_____ Any lumps or tenderness in axilla?

_____ Any skin irritation?

Genitourinary

_____ Pain in kidney region?

_____ Get up at night to urinate? How many times? _____

_____ Swelling of hands or feet?

In the evening? _____

In the morning? _____

_____ Blood or pus in urine?

_____ Albumin in urine?

_____ Sugar in urine?

_____ Frequent urination?

_____ Burning or pain on urination?

_____ Pain over bladder?

_____ Trouble starting urine?

_____ Urinary stream weak?

_____ Hard to empty bladder completely?

_____ Hard to control urine when coughing or sneezing?

_____ History of stones?

_____ Sexually active?

_____ Method of contraception?

_____

_____ Any sexual concerns?

_____ History of venereal disease?

Males

_____ Any discharge, irritation, or lesion?

_____ Any scrotal pain or swelling?

_____ Any tenderness or enlargement of prostate?

_____ Any hernias?

Females

_____ Menses:

> Date of last period?_____
>
> Age menses began? _____
>
> Now occurs about every ____ days
>
> Number of days of flow? ____
>
> Flooding? Number of pads per day _____

_____ Irregular?

_____ Painful?

_____ Spotting between periods?

_____ Age when "change of life" started? _____

_____ Hot flashes?

_____ Any history of trouble with female organs?

_____ Pregnancies? Number? _____

_____ Complications of pregnancy?

_____ Any miscarriages?

_____ Vaginal itching?

_____ Increase in amount of vaginal discharge?

_____ Taken antibiotics in past month?

_____ Taking birth control pill?

_____ Date of last Pap smear?

Musculoskeletal

_____ Poor coordination?

_____ Swollen or painful joints?

_____ Stiffness of muscles or joints?

_____ Muscle cramps in arms or legs?

_____ Painful feet or hands?

_____ Backache?

_____ Pain or stiffness in neck?

_____ Muscle weakness or twitching?

_____ Sprain or fracture?

_____ Difficulty with feeding self, dressing, walking?

Neurological

_____ Headaches?

_____ Dizziness or fainting?

_____ Drowsiness?

_____ Loss of consciousness?

_____ Seizures or convulsions?

_____ Numbness, tingling, or de-creased sensation?

_____ Twitching muscles?

_____ Muscle weakness or paralysis?

_____ Clumsy or have frequent acci-dents?

_____ Unsteady? Shaky?

_____ Forgetful? Loss of memory?

_____ History of head trauma?

_____ Delayed growth and develop-ment?

Psychosocial

_____ From a nervous family?

_____ Considered to be a nervous person?

_____ Tremble and sweat easily?

_____ Have trouble making up your mind?

_____ Easily mixed-up or confused?

_____ Feel sad, lonely, or depressed?

_____ Cry often?

_____ Wish you were dead?

_____ Worry continually?

_____ Upset by little things?

_____ A perfectionist?

_____ Often misunderstood?

_____ Often act on sudden impulse?

_____ Easily angered?

_____ Frequently keyed-up and jittery?

_____ Bites your nails?

_____ Easily scared by sudden noises?

_____ Have bad thoughts or dreams?

_____ Have trouble getting along with
someone at home, school, or
work?

_____ Under a lot of pressure?

Social history

Marital status _____

Composition of family _____

Roles and responsibilities of family members _____

_____

Occupation _____

Economic status _____

Housing _____

Dietary patterns

   Typical daily meal plan _____

   _____

   _____

   Dietary restrictions _____

   Fluid intake _____

Habits

Number of cigarettes per day?	_____	Number of Cokes per day?	_____
Other tobacco per day?	_____	Alcoholic drinks per day?	_____
Cups of coffee per day?	_____	Use of drugs?	_____

Resting patterns

   Hours worked per day? _____

   Hours sleep per night? _____

   Rest periods or naps? _____

Description of activities in typical day _____

_____

_____

Exercise pattern

    Amount of exercise per day? _____

    Restrictions?_____

Recreation and hobbies _____

Education _____

Cultural background _____

Religion _____

Behavior during assessment_____

Ability to understand English _____

Reliability of data given _____

APPENDIX 2

MODEL ADULT PHYSICAL ASSESSMENT FORM

Vital Statistics:

Temp _____ Pulse _____ Resp _____ Height _____ Weight _____

Blood Pressure: Sitting _____ Standing _____ Supine _____

Check (✔) if normal, *NE* if not examined, *X* if abnormal. Describe abnormal findings.

General overview   Description

_____ Normal posture, stature, gait

_____ No involuntary movements

_____ Articulates well, no speech impediments

_____ Facial appearance _____

_____ Neat and well-groomed

_____ Nutritional status_____

_____ Growth and development appropriate for age

_____ Well-oriented

_____ Cooperative

Skin

_____ Color _____

_____ Warm and dry

_____ Good turgor

_____ No lesions or rashes

_____ No varicosities

_____ No vascular or purpuric lesions

_____ No swelling or edema

_____ No body odor

Nails

_____ No cyanosis of nail beds

_____ Angle at base of nail approximately 160°, no clubbing

_____ Rapid capillary filling

Hair

_____ Color _____

_____ Texture _____

_____ Amount _____

_____ Distribution _____

_____ No foreign material

_____ No lesions on scalp

_____ No dandruff or scaling of scalp

Head and face

_____ Normocephalic, symmetrical

_____ No lumps or tenderness

_____ Facial nerve (N.VII): Symmetrical, movement intact

_____ Trigeminal nerve (N.V): Motor and sensory, all three divisions intact

_____ TM joint freely movable, no pain

Neck

_____ Full ROM

_____ Spinal accessory (N.XI): intact, strong

_____ Trachea in midline

_____ Thyroid: Nonpalpable, no masses

_____ Salivary glands, Nontender,
not enlarged

_____ Carotid pulses 4 + , equal

_____ Lymph nodes: No enlargement
or tenderness

    _____ Preauricular

    _____ Postauricular

    _____ Occipital

    _____ Tonsillar

    _____ Submandibular

    _____ Submental

    _____ Anterior cervical

    _____ Posterior cervical

    _____ Supraclavicular

    _____ Infraclavicular

Eyes

_____ Eyes, brows, and lids: Good
alignment, symmetrical

_____ Lids: No lid lag, no inflammation

_____ Sclera: White

_____ Conjunctiva: Pink, noninflamed

_____ Lacrimal glands: Nontender

_____ Iris: Round, intact

_____ PERRLA

_____ Normal visual fields (N.II)

_____ Convergence within 5 to 8 cm

_____ Extraocular movements intact
(N.III, IV, VI)

_____ Visual acuity:

    Corrected:
        OD_____ OS_____
    Uncorrected:
        OD_____ OS_____

_____ Corneal reflex intact (N.V)

_____ Cornea, lens: No opacities

Fundi

_____ Optic disks: Flat, yellow, margins clear

_____ Physiologic cup flat

_____ Arteries, veins: Normal ratio

_____ No AV nicking, hemorrhage or exudate

Ears

_____ Symmetrical

_____ Correct alignment with eyes

_____ Auricle: No masses or tenderness

_____ Canal: No lesions or discharge, cerumen present

_____ Tympanic membrane: Clear, intact, good light reflex, all landmarks present

_____ Auditory acuity (N.VIII) normal to ticking watch or whisper

_____ Weber: lateralizes equally

_____ Rinne: AC is greater than BC

Nose and sinuses

_____ Mucosa and turbinates: Pink, no discharge, polyps, or edema

_____ Septum: No deviation

_____ Patent bilaterally

_____ Sinuses: Nontender

    _____ Frontal

    _____ Maxillary

Mouth and pharynx

_____ Lips: No lesions or edema

_____ Teeth and gums: In good repair, no obvious caries, no bleeding or edema

_____ Mucous membrane: Pink, no lesions

_____ Tonsils: No crypts, enlargement, redness, or exudate

_____ Salivary ducts: no edema
or redness

_____ Tongue: Pink, no lesions, fasciculations, or asymmetry
(N.XII)

_____ Gag reflex present (N.IX, X)

_____ Soft palate and uvula rise
equally (N.IX, X)

Thorax and lungs

_____ Thorax symmetrical, no
deformity

_____ Respiration: Regular rhythm

_____ Rate of respirations _____

_____ Respiratory expansion symmetrical

_____ Diaphragmatic excursion 3 to
5 cm

_____ Fremitus equal, bilateral

_____ Lungs resonant

_____ Breath sounds normal

    _____ Vesicular: Inspiration
is greater than expira-
tion

    _____ Bronchovesicular: In-
spiration is equal to ex-
piration

    _____ Bronchial: Inspiration
is less than expiration

    _____ No rales, rhonchi,
wheezes, or rubs

Breasts and axillae

_____ Size _____

_____ Symmetrical

_____ Smooth contour, no dimpling
or flattening

_____ No masses or tenderness

_____ Nipples erect, no discharge

_____ No gynecomastia (male)

_____ Instructed in BSE

_____ Axillary lymph nodes: No enlargement or tenderness

     _____ Lateral

     _____ Central

     _____ Pectoral (anterior)

     _____ Subscapular (posterior)

Heart

_____ PMI left midclavicular

_____ No thrills or abnormal pulsations

_____ Regular sinus rhythm, rate _____

_____ Aortic-pulmonic: S_2 is greater than S_1, no murmurs or rubs

_____ Tricuspid-mitral: S_1 is greater than S_2, no murmurs or rubs, no S_3 or S_4

Peripheral vascular

_____ Jugular venous pressure is less than 3 cm above sternal angle

_____ Carotid pulses: 4+ (on 0 to 4 scale), symmetrical

_____ Arms and hands: Skin and nail beds pink, smooth, warm, and dry

_____ No clubbing or edema

_____ Radial, ulnar, and brachial pulses 4+

_____ Legs and feet: Skin and nail beds pink, smooth, warm, and dry

_____ No pretibial, ankle, or hand edema

_____ No varicosities or ulceration

_____ Homans' sign negative, no calf tenderness

_____ Femoral, popliteal, posterior tibial and dorsalis pedis pulses 4+

_____ Epitrochlear and inguinal nodes nonpalpable, nontender

Abdomen

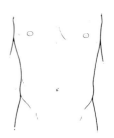

_____ Skin: No scars, striae, rashes, lesions, or dilated veins

_____ Umbilicus: Normal contour, no herniation, contour _____

_____ No distention, rigidity, or ascites

_____ Liver size within 6 to 12 cm midclavicular

_____ Bowel sounds present, no hyperactivity

_____ No bruits or friction rubs

_____ Light palpation: No masses or tenderness

_____ Deep palpation: No masses, tenderness, or rebound tenderness

_____ Liver, spleen, kidneys nonpalpable, nontender

_____ No inguinal or femoral herniation

Musculoskeletal

_____ TM joint: No swelling, tenderness, or crepitation

Neck

_____ Full ROM

_____ No joint deformity, swelling, or tenderness

_____ Normal muscle strength

Hands and wrists

_____ Full ROM

_____ No swelling, nodules, or bony enlargement

_____ No deformity or atrophy

_____ Muscle strength normal, symmetrical

Elbows

_____ Full ROM, no nodules, tenderness, or swelling

Shoulders

_____ Full ROM

_____ No swelling, deformity, or atrophy

_____ No tenderness or crepitation

_____ Normal muscle strength

Thorax

_____ No swelling or tenderness of costochondral junctions

_____ Rib cage symmetrical

_____ Ribs intact

_____ Clavicles intact

Feet and ankles

_____ Full ROM

_____ No deformities or nodules

_____ No calluses, corns, or bony enlargement

_____ No tenderness or swelling/fluid

_____ Normal muscle strength

Knees and hips

_____ Full ROM

_____ Normal muscle strength

_____ No deformity, crepitus, fluid, tenderness, atrophy, or bony enlargement

Spine

_____ No scoliosis, lordosis, or kyphosis

_____ No tenderness or spasm of paravertebral and trapezius muscles

_____ No tenderness of spine

_____ Full ROM

_____ No pain on straight-leg lifting

_____ Performs normal activities of daily living

Neurological (Items marked with an asterisk (*) are to be checked on all clients; others are to be checked as indicated.)

Cranial nerves

_____ N.I: Correctly identifies odors

_____ *N.II: Normal visual fields

 _____ Visual acuity corrected

 OD _____ OS _____

 _____ Optic disks: Within normal limits

_____ *N.III: PERRLA

 _____ EOM intact

 _____ No ptosis or lid lag

_____ N.IV: Downward medial movement of eyes intact

_____ N.V: Sensory perception of pain, light touch, temperature, intact in ophthalmic, maxillary and mandibular division

 _____ Motor function strong with clenched teeth

 _____ Corneal reflexes present

_____ N.VI: Lateral deviation of eye intact

 _____ No nystagmus

_____ N.VII: Facial muscles strong and symmetrical

 _____ Taste present on anterior tongue

_____ *N.VIII: Auditory acuity normal to ticking watch or whisper

 _____ AC is greater than BC (Rinne)

 _____ No lateralization (Weber)

_____ N.IX, N.X: Normal gag reflex

    _____ Soft palate and uvula symmetrical with upward movement

    _____ Taste present on posterior tongue

_____ N.XI: Sternocleidomastoids and trapezii muscles strong, symmetrical

_____ N.XII: Tongue symmetrical, no deviation, atrophy, or fasciculation

Motor

_____ *Normal gait, heel-to-toe, deep knee bends, walking on heels and toes

_____ *Romberg negative

_____ Good coordination: Finger-to-nose, patting leg, heel-to-shin

_____ Grip strong, no tremor or drift of arms

_____ Muscles: no atrophy, fasciculations, involuntary movements, or abnormal positions

_____ Muscles firm, strong, symmetrical strength

Sensory

_____ *Pain perception intact

_____ Perception of light touch, temperature, and vibration intact

_____ Normal position sense and point discrimination

_____ Normal stereognosis and number identification

Mental status and speech

_____ *Orientation to person, place, time

_____ Recent and remote memory good

_____ Serial 7s, 3s normal

_____ Able to abstract

_____ Dress and behavior appropriate

_____ Mood_____

Reflexes (on 0 to 4 scale, normal is 2 +)

_____ *Biceps (C_5, C_6)

_____ *Triceps (C_7, C_8)

_____ *Brachioradialis (C_5, C_6)

_____ Abdominal (T_8, T_9, $T_{10}\downarrow$, T_{10} T_{11}, $T_{12}\downarrow$)

_____ Cremasteric (L_1, L_2)

_____ *Patellar (L_2, L_3, L_4)

_____ *Achilles (S_1, S_2)

_____ Plantar (L_4, L_5, S_1, S_2)

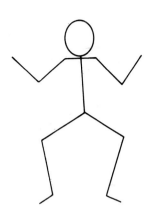

Male genitalia

_____ Penis: Circumcised

    _____ No discharge, inflammation, or swelling

    _____ No ulcers, scars, or nodules

    _____ Urethral meatus correct location

_____ Scrotum: No masses, ulceration, or lesions

    _____ No inflammation or edema of scrotum

_____ Testes and epididymis: Normal size and consistency

_____ No inguinal or femoral hernia

_____ Prostate: Soft, nontender, no enlargement or nodules

Female genitalia and pelvis

_____ Vulva: No inflammation or edema, no tenderness or masses

_____ Vagina: Mucosa pink, no lesions, moist, no excessive discharge

_____ Vaginal outlet: Good muscle tone, no bulging of mucosa

_____ Urethra: No inflammation or discharge

_____ Cervix: Position normal, no lesions, nodules, or ulcerations, no bleeding or discharge

_____ Uterus: Anterior, midline, smooth, not enlarged

_____ Adnexae: Ovaries normal size and consistency, nontender

_____ Rectovaginal exam: No masses

_____ Pap smear: _____

Rectum and anus

_____ No inflammation, rash, or excoriation

_____ No lesions, fissures, or hemorrhoids

_____ No masses

_____ Sphincter tone good

_____ No bleeding

_____ No pilonidal cyst

_____ Stool _____

APPENDIX 3

NEWBORN ASSESSMENT GUIDE

The information needed to adequately assess the health status of the newborn and infant is sufficiently different to warrant a separate tool. At times, special techniques and approaches must be used by the examiner to complete an accurate examination of the newborn or infant. Such an examination is essential in determining the newborn and infant adjustment and response to the extrauterine environment and as baseline data for the child health record.

In the preceding modules, you will note that information has been given under the pediatric adaptations of the physical and history, and Posttest questions have been asked in relation to the examination and findings on the newborn and infant. However, health assessments are frequently required on these young clients in the newborn nursery, pediatrician's office, and community health home and clinic visits; the authors felt a separate history and physical examination tool would be of assistance to you.

You will also note that suggested references are given for examination of this type of client. For more detailed information, the student may wish to review the suggested references and Decision Tables within each module.

The key to examining the newborn and infant is in handling these small clients in such a way that the data obtained are reliable. The parents' cooperation is often most helpful, and with proper instruction they may prove willing assistants.

Client cooperation is nonexistent, but keeping the infant warm and supplying a nipple will often keep the infant quiet long enough to complete the examination. Instead of proceeding with a cephalocaudal examination, it is often wise to begin with general observations and then listen to the chest while the infant is quiet. Head and neck may be left for last since these may cause discomfort.

Suggested References

Mc Millan, Julia, and Phillip I. Nieburg: *Whole Pediatrician Catalog,* Saunders, Philadelphia, 1977 (newborn chapter).

Korones, Sheldon: *High Risk Newborn Infants,* Mosby, St. Louis, 1976, pp. 53-58, 100-121.

Barness, Lewis A.: *Manual of Pediatric Physical Diagnosis,* Year Book, Chicago, 1972, pp. 179-210.

Alexander, Mary M., and Marie Scott Brown: *Pediatric History Taking and Physical Diagnosis for Nurses,* McGraw-Hill, New York, 1979, pp. 376-381.

History of Newborn Infant

Name _____ Age _____ Sex _____

Ethnic origin _____ Residence _____

Occupation of parents_____

Education of parents _____ Religion of parents _____

Number, sex, and age of other persons in family:

Relationship	Age	Sex	Health

Past history

1. Diet of mother during pregnancy?_____

2. Health of mother during pregnancy? _____

3. X-rays of mother during pregnancy? _____

4. Blood type of mother? _____ Blood type of father? _____

5. Presence of bleeding? _____

6. Drugs during pregnancy: Prescription _____

   Nonprescription _____

   Other (LSD, marijuana, heroin, etc.) _____

7. Length of pregnancy? _____ months

8. Duration of labor?_____

9. Type of delivery? _____

10. Type of analgesia or anesthesia?_____

11. Place of birth? _____

12. Infant's condition at birth? _____ 5-min Apgar score _____

    a. Cry, color, breathing _____

    b. Birth weight _____

13. Neonatal complications:

    a. Jaundice (before or after 48 hours) _____

    b. Cyanosis _____

    c. Convulsions _____

    d. Deformities _____

    e. Other _____

14. Nutrition:

    a. Number of feedings per day _____

    b. Formula (kind and preparation) _____

    c. Quantity of formula taken _____

    d. Breast (length of feeding at each breast) _____

    e. Appetite _____

    f. Tolerance of feedings (vomiting, diarrhea) _____

    g. Approximate calories per day _____

    h. Amount and kinds of fluids per day (juice, water, etc.) _____

    i. Age at introduction to solid food _____

        (1) Method of introduction _____

        (2) Amount of solids currently taken (cereal, egg, vegetables, fruits, meats)

        _____

        (3) Typical diet for one day _____

        _____

        (4) Eating between meals _____

        (5) Likes and dislikes _____

        (6) Vitamins (dosage per day) _____

15. Sleep pattern (quiet, restless) _____

    a. Length of sleep at night _____

    b. Number and lengths of naps _____

    c. Average number of times infant wakens during night _____

16. Elimination:

   a. Stools

      (1) Number per day _____   (4) Constipation _____

      (2) Color and consistency _____   (5) Difficulty _____

      (3) Odor _____   (6) Age of bowel control _____

   b. Urine voidings

      (1) Number per day _____   (4) Crying with urination _____

      (2) Color and odor _____   (5) Age of bladder control _____

      (3) Difficulty passing _____

17. Disposition/behavior:

   a. Happy_____   d. Thumb-sucking _____

   b. Fussy _____   e. Tics _____

   c. Sleepy _____   f. Tantrums _____

18. Immunization record:

   a. DPT _____   d. Polio_____

   b. Measles _____   e. TB _____

   c. Mumps_____   f. Smallpox _____

Infant Development (age achieved)

1. Held up head _____   4. Spoke single word _____

2. Sat alone _____   5. Weaned _____

3. Stood alone _____   6. Age first tooth _____

4. Walked alone _____

Previous illness

1. General health _____

2. Previous hospitalizations (duration, diagnosis, name of hospital) _____

   _____

3. Contagious diseases:

	Age	Symptoms	Diagnostic criteria	Complications
a.				
b.				
c.				
d.				

4. Allergies: _____

   a. Urticaria _____   d. Hay fever _____

   b. Eczema _____   e. Drug sensitivities _____

   c. Asthma _____

5. Accidents and operations (burns, poisoning, head trauma, fractures) _____

   _____

History of present illness

Events pertinent to present health status:

1. Time factor regarding symptoms _____

2. Description of earliest to present symptoms _____

3. Aggravating factors _____

4. Alleviating factors_____

5. Consultations for complaint _____

6. Medical diagnosis _____

7. Treatment _____

8. Medications given and amount_____

9. Complications _____

10. Effect of illness on infant's activity, appetite, weight, temperature, quality of cry

    _____

    _____

Review of Systems

(Select items relevant to client's age and development which have not already been covered.)

If the answer is *yes,* place a check (✔) at the left and provide further information in the Remarks column.

General overview   Remarks

_____ General health
_____ Lost or gained weight (amount)
_____ Difficulty sleeping or going to sleep
_____ Chills, fever
_____ Lethargy, extreme activity
_____ Convulsions
_____ Change in quality of cry
_____ Hoarseness at times

Skin

_____ Any skin diseases
_____ Rashes
_____ Swelling or lumps
_____ Dry skin
_____ Excessive sweating
_____ Change in color or pigmentation
_____ Tenderness
_____ Recent loss of hair
_____ Change in hair growth
_____ Color changes in nails or lips
_____ Sores on body

Head and neck

_____ Rubs head
_____ Sleeps with head on same side
_____ Head injury
_____ Stiffness in neck
_____ Decreased movement
_____ Swelling or enlarged glands
_____ Development of or changes in head control

Eyes

_____ Redness or discharge

_____ Crossing

_____ Infection

_____ Rubbing eyes

_____ Tearing

Ears

_____ Turns to noise

_____ Rubs or pulls at ears

_____ Discharge

_____ Earaches

_____ Loss of balance

_____ Foreign bodies in ears

Nose and sinuses

_____ Frequent stuffy or runny nose

_____ Nosebleeds

_____ Breathes through nose

_____ Rubs at nose or face

_____ Frequent use of nose drops

_____ Foreign bodies in nose

Mouth and throat

_____ Frequent colds or sore throat

_____ Sore mouth or throat

_____ Change in color or coating of tongue

_____ Teething behavior (fever, pain, fussiness, etc.)

Gastrointestinal

_____ Poor appetite

_____ Nausea or vomiting

_____ Vomiting of blood

_____ Gas

_____ Yellow skin or eyes

_____ Difficulty swallowing

_____ Draws knees up and cries

_____ Diarrhea

_____ Constipation
_____ Black or tarry stools
_____ Mucus in stools
_____ Uses laxatives or enemas
_____ Colic
_____ Change in number of stools
_____ Change in quality of suck

Cardiovascular and pulmonary

_____ Heart pounds or races
_____ Color change during feeding
_____ Difficulty breathing during
feeding
_____ Has a heart murmur
_____ Turns blue around mouth or
nails
_____ Coughs up sputum or blood
_____ Recent or chronic cough
_____ Wheezing or grunting with
respirations
_____ Difficulty breathing
_____ Swelling of eyes, hands, feet
_____ Two-tone cry
_____ Noisy respirations
_____ Retractions
_____ Head-rocking with breathing
_____ Sweating
_____ Head must be elevated to sleep

Breast and axilla

_____ Nipple discharge
_____ Enlargement, tenderness,
lumps

Genitourinary

_____ Blood or pus in diaper
_____ Frequent urination or defeca-
tion
_____ Crying with elimination

Males

_____ Discharge, irritation, lesion
_____ Scrotal swelling
_____ Scrotal discoloration
_____ Hernias

Females

_____ Redness of labia
_____ Vaginal discharge
_____ Lesions

Musculoskeletal

_____ Swollen, painful joints
_____ Stiffness in muscles, joints
_____ Muscle weakness
_____ Fractures/injuries
_____ Muscle twitching

Neurological

_____ Limpness, lethargy
_____ Extreme irritability
_____ Bulging, tense fontanels
_____ Sunken fontanels
_____ Seizures/convulsions
_____ Paralysis

Family History

1. Parents married _____

2. Age and health or date and cause of death of:

   Father _____ Mother _____

3. Other pregnancies:

Pregnancy complications	Type of delivery	Miscarriages	Neonatal complications

4. Present or recent contagious diseases in family: _____

5. Familial disease (describe those present):

Tuberculosis _____   Mental illness _____

Allergy _____   Blood disease_____

Diabetes _____   Congenital malformations _____

Cardiac disease _____   Infections _____

Renal disease_____   Cancer _____

Neurologic disease _____   Trauma _____

6. Developmental (If infant has delayed development, obtain history of development of both parents — see Infant Development, above). _____

7. Parental use of alcohol, drugs _____

8. Maturity of parents _____

Social history

1. Nearness of relatives _____

2. Approximate financial status _____

3. Home conditions:

    a. Number of people_____

    b. Number of bedrooms _____

    c. Sleeping arrangements _____

    d. Number of bathrooms_____

    e. Pets _____

    f. Source of water and milk supply_____

    g. Kitchen facilities (refrigerator, stove, etc.)_____

4. Recreational activity of parents_____

5. Parental activity with other couples, friends _____

6. Babysitting arrangements _____

7. Psychosocial: **Father**   **Mother**

    a. From nervous family

    b. Considered to be nervous

    c. Cries often

    d. Easily upset or confused

    e. Under a lot of pressure

    f. Trembles or sweats easily

    g. Easily angered

    h. Worries continually

    i. Perfectionistic

    j. Feels sad, lonely, or depressed

Physical Assessment of Newborn/ Infant

Child's name _____ Date _____

General information

Date and hour of birth _____ Age at exam _____

Apgar score: 1 min _____ 5 min _____ Entry into nursery _____

Gestational age: By history _____ By physical assessment _____

Length of labor _____ Type of delivery _____

Birth length _____ Current length _____ Birth weight _____

Current weight _____ Temperature _____ Pulse _____

Respiration _____ Blood pressure _____

Head circumference at birth _____

Check (✔) if normal, mark *NE* if not examined, and *X* if abnormal. Describe all abnormal findings.

Overview appraisal   Description

_____ Symmetry/body proportion

_____ Position/posture

_____ Activity level/responsiveness

_____ Quality of cry (description)

Skin

_____ Color

_____ Pigmentation

_____ Texture/turgor

_____ Wrinkles/peeling

_____ Lanugo/vernix

_____ Milia

_____ Opacity/translucency

_____ Hair distribution

_____ Lymph nodes (hypertrophy— local, general, consistency, tenderness, adherence to nearby structures)

_____ Mucous membranes (dry, pale, pink)

Head

_____ Circumference

_____ Shape/symmetry

_____ Contours/molding

_____ Fontanels

       _____ Anterior size, tension, pulsations

       _____ Posterior size

       _____ Extra fontanels

_____ Suture size

_____ Movement, head lag

_____ Hair distribution, amount

       _____ Texture (fine, electric)

       _____ Whorls

_____ Scalp condition

Face

_____ Shape, symmetry

_____ Expression

_____ Movement symmetry

_____ Nasolabial fold, depth and length

_____ Jaw size, movement

_____ Chin distance from lips

Eyes

_____ Placement, symmetry

_____ Inner canthal distance

_____ Size, slant

_____ Cornea clarity, luster

_____ Blink reflex

_____ Pupil size, reaction, position

_____ Color of sclera

_____ Color of conjunctiva

_____ Muscular control

_____ Discharge, tearing

_____ Placement and shape of eyebrows

_____ Eyelids, lashes

_____ Lens, opacity

Nose

_____ Shape, placement

_____ External appearance

_____ Breadth of bridge

_____ Patency

_____ Septum

_____ Discharge

_____ Movement of nares/flaring

Mouth

_____ Shape, placement

_____ Size, symmetry

_____ Shape, arch of hard palate

_____ Soft palate, uvula

_____ Color of mucosa, gums

_____ Tonsil size

_____ Pharynx (color, edema)

_____ Teeth (quality, number)

_____ Salivation

_____ Quality of suck

_____ Rooting reflex

_____ Tongue size

    _____ Grooves, creases

    _____ Color, coating

    _____ Movement (fasciculations)

Ears

_____ Alignment with eyes

_____ Shape, symmetry

_____ Rotation

_____ Development, firmness

_____ Pinna size, position

_____ Adherent lobes

_____ Tympanic membrane

_____ Hearing acuity

Neck

_____ Size (circumference and length)

_____ Thyroid (palpation, position, contour)

_____ Masses, nodes

_____ Flexion, movement

_____ Carotid pulses, venous distribution

_____ Bruits, thrills

_____ Position of trachea

Chest

_____ Circumference

_____ Shape, symmetry

_____ Movement, retractions

_____ Sternum length, width

_____ Axillary masses

_____ Lungs

    _____ Percussion (dullness)

    _____ Breath sounds

    _____ Depth respiration

    _____ Rate, regularity of respiration

    _____ Palpable thrills

    _____ Fremitus

_____ Rachitic rosary beads
_____ Apex heart/PMI
    _____ Heart rate, rhythm
    _____ Heart sounds
_____ Nipple position, symmetry
    _____ Size
    _____ Distance between

Abdomen
_____ Size, contour
_____ Musculature, masses
_____ Tension, pulsations
_____ Umbilical cord, hernia
_____ Inguinal hernia
_____ Palpation of liver, spleen, kidneys
_____ Rectal patency, discharge
_____ Shifting dullness, fluid waves
_____ Visible peristalsis

Genitalia
Female
_____ Labia size, symmetry
_____ Secretions, discharge
_____ Lesions
Male
_____ Foreskin, circumcision
_____ Meatal opening
_____ Scrotum size, color
_____ Testes descended
_____ Secretions, discharge
_____ Lesions

Musculoskeletal
_____ Hips
    _____ Movement, flexion, clicks
    _____ Symmetry
    _____ Gluteal folds even
    _____ Equal hip-to-knee lengths

_____ Extremities
      _____ Range of motion
      _____ Length, symmetry
      _____ Movement, tremors
      _____ Pulses
      _____ Number of digits
      _____ Nail quality
      _____ Dermatoglyphics
_____ Back and spine
      _____ Movement, symmetry
      _____ Posture
      _____ Curvatures
      _____ Alignment of scapulae

Reflexes

Early infancy and newborn

_____ Grasp up to 4 months
_____ Stepping up to 4 months
_____ Tonic neck up to 6 months
_____ Babinski positive until 12 months
_____ Moro up to 6 months
_____ Swallowing, gagging

Later infancy

_____ Landau
_____ Parachute

Landau —
Parachute —

Lab data

_____ CBC
_____ Hgb
_____ Hct
_____ PKU result
_____ T_4 result

PRETEST ANSWERS

Module 1

1. a. Establishing and maintaining a professional-client relationship
    b. Listening to allow client to express feelings
    c. Obtaining information which allows for the identification of health care needs
    d. Giving information
    e. Educating client
    f. Counseling client
    g. Referral of client to additional sources for care
2. a. Courteous treatment of client
    b. Making client as comfortable as possible before beginning interview
    c. Providing for geographical and psychological privacy
    d. Providing freedom from interruption during interview
    e. Conveying an attitude of emotional objectivity
    f. Implementation of attentive listening skills on the part of the interviewer
3. a. I   b. T   c. P   d. I   e. D   f. T   g. I   h. P   i. I   j. T
4. a. Reassuring (c)
    b. Probing (d)
    c. Understanding (e)
    d. Evaluative (a)
    e. Hostile (b)
5. Blocks to effective communication
6. True
7. False. Data are collected using all senses.
8. False. Assessment of both verbal and nonverbal behavior is essential.

9. False. Nonverbal behavior most often occurs out of the conscious awareness of the client.

10. True

11. True

12. True

13. False. Silence often indicates acceptance and gives the client time to think through and formulate a response.

14. True

15. False. Interviewer will support and encourage the client to share feelings.

16. False. Allowing the client to cry indicates that the interviewer is comfortable in the interaction and can accept the patient's feelings.

17. True

18. True

19. True

20. False. Clients often attempt to handle health problems themselves, or seek the aid of a friend or relative prior to seeking medical attention.

21. False. The interviewer's expectations have the same degree of influence as the client's.

22. False. The best interview situation occurs when the client and interviewer can freely interact.

23. False. The good interviewer always encourages the client to accept responsibility for the client's own feelings, actions, and health care decisions.

24. False. A helping interview is usually unstructured and guided by the client's needs.

25. False. The information-getting interview is highly structured.

26. False. The interviewer brings his or her own set of personal biases and beliefs to the interview which cause the interviewer to turn a blind eye to certain phases of the discussion.

27. True

28. False. Both parent and child should be consulted.

29. True

30. True

31. False. Each interviewer establishes his or her own relationship with the client. Depending upon the quality of that relationship, information will vary.

32. True

33. True

34. False. Adolescents are uncomfortable in social relationships and long silences may make them feel awkward and hopelessly uncomfortable.

35. True

36. True

37. True

38. False. Information is constantly collected over the lifetime of the relationship.

39. a. The client may not understand the interviewer.

    b. When the client does not understand the interviewer, the interviewer tends to become increasingly irritated.

    c. Sick-role behaviors may differ from that of the white, urban, educated middle- and upper-class norm and thus be misunderstood by the professional.

    d. Client may need to deny or ignore illness for as long as possible to reduce economic or social loss. Preventive health measures may be unknown.

    e. The effect of social distance may cause client to adopt a posture of outward compliance or subservience which disguises distrust.

f. Lack of coordination and continuity of health care may leave the client confused, angry, frightened, and distrustful of health professionals.

g. Differences in social class may convince the client that it is impossible to be truly understood by middle- and upper-class professionals.

40. a. Not helpful. Interviewer should face client and speak slowly, clearly, and with a low tone of voice.

b. Helpful

c. Not helpful. This is a need of the elderly person. The nurse should be supportive unless the person withdraws into the past.

d. Not helpful. This is degrading.

e. Not helpful. Client may have impairment of memory or some neurological changes that would go unidentified without a system of cross-checks.

Module 3

1. a. Production of vitamin D

b. Protection of deeper tissues from injury and invasion

c. Protection of deeper tissues from drying

d. Assists in regulation of body temperature

e. Serves as an organ of excretion

f. Supports peripheral nerve endings

2. See anatomy textbook.

3. a. Apocrine sweat gland

b. Hair shaft

c. Hair bulb

d. Hair follicle

e. Sebaceous gland

f. Body of eccrine gland

g. Pore of eccrine gland

h. Duct of eccrine gland

i. Stratum corneum of epidermis (horny layer)

j. Stratum mucosum of epidermis (cellular layer)

k. Fat cells

l. Blood vessels

m. Ridge

n. Furrow

4. a. Free margin of nail

b. Nail fold

c. Nail sulcus

d. Nail plate

e. Lunula

f. Cuticle

g. Eponychium

5. True

6. False. The epidermis is uniformly thin over the whole body, but measures 0.06 to 0.1 mm. Total skin thickness may vary from 1.5 to 4 mm.

7. True

8. False. The epidermis is replaced about every 28 days.
9. True
10. True
11. False. The chief components of sweat are water, sodium, potassium, chloride, glucose, urea, and lactate.
12. True
13. True
14. False. Body odor is caused by bacterial decomposition of apocrine sweat.
15. False. Sebum is secreted by the sebaceous glands.
16. False. The activity of sebaceous glands is increased by androgens and limited by the production of estrogens.
17. True
18. True
19. False. The major function of the dermis is to provide nutrition for the epidermis.
20. True
21. True
22. False. The skin normally harbors pseudomonas, group A hemolytic streptococci, nonhemolytic streptococci, diphtherids, mycobacteria, and coagulase positive and negative staphlococci.
23. False. The normal pH is 4.2 to 5.6.
24. a
25. c
26. b

Module 4

1 and 2. See anatomy book.
3.

II	c	1
III	b	4, 5, 6
IV	e	3
V	d	7
VI	a	2

Module 5

1 and 2. See anatomy textbook.
3. Acoustic nerve (VIII)
4. Transmit sound waves from the tympanic membrane to the oval window of the inner ear
5. Hearing, balance

Module 6

1 to 7. See anatomy textbook.
8.

I	d	5
V	f	1, 6, 11
VII	a	3, 7
XI	b	8
X	g	4, 9
XI	e	10
XII	c	2

Module 7

1. See anatomy textbook.
2. See anatomy textbook.
3. a. 1 through 7
   b. 8 through 10
   c. 11 through 12
4. f   d   h   j   g   e   a   c   b   i
5. Respiration is composed of two processes, inspiration and expiration. The purpose of respiration is to exchange gases from the air into the blood stream and vice versa.
6. Eupnea
7. 1 to 4 – one respiration to every four heartbeats
8. a. Newborn: 30 to 50
   b. 6-month-old to 2-year-old: 20 to 30
   c. Adolescent: 12 to 30
   d. Adult: 16 to 20
9. a. Exercise
   b. Body temperature
   c. Age
   d. State of hydration
   e. Anxiety
   f. Altitude
10. True
11. False. The diaphragm returns to its original position, increasing the pressure in the thoracic cage.
12. False. The left lung has no middle lobe. The right middle lobe of the lung underlies the right anterior and lateral thorax.
13. True
14. True
15. True
16. True
17. True
18. False. Intercostales interni decrease the size of the thoracic cavity.
19. True
20. True
21. False. It decreases the acidity of the blood.
22. True
23. True
24. False. A constant negative interpleural pressure is necessary for normal respirations.
25. False. The major innervation for the diaphragm is the phrenic nerve.
26. True
27. False. Bronchioles are less than 1 mm in diameter and have no connective tissue sheath.
28. True
29. True
30. True
31. g
32. a

33. j
34. e
35. d
36. b
37. c
38. h
39. i
40. f
41. a, e
42. d
43. f
44. e
45. e, d

Module 8

1. a. Pulmonary capillary
    b. Pulmonary artery
    c. Superior vena cava
    d. Pulmonic valve
    e. Right atrium
    f. Tricuspid valve
    g. Inferior vena cava
    h. Right ventricle
    i. Left ventricle
    j. Mitral valve
    k. Aortic valve
    l. Left atrium
    m. Pulmonary vein
    n. Aorta
    o. Alveolus of lung

2. a. Lungs
    b. Pulmonary vein
    c. Left atrium
    d. Left ventricle
    e. Aorta
    f. Left subclavian
    g. Left brachioradialis artery

3. a. Cardiac output
    b. Elastic recoil blood vessels
    c. Peripheral resistance
    d. Volume of blood
    e. Viscosity of blood

4. Peripheral resistance of blood vessels
5. See anatomy textbook.
6. Middle
7. See anatomy textbook.

Module 9

1 to 3. See anatomy textbook.
4. b
5. There are many functions. A few are production of bile; carbohydrate, fat, and protein metabolism; detoxification of substances; storage of vitamins A, B, B_{12}, and iron; phagocytosis; formation of heparin.
6. a. Concentration of bile
    b. Storage of bile
7. Digests fats; emulsifies fats; absorbs fatty acids
8. Bilirubin, jaundice

Module 11

1. See anatomy textbook.
2. 5 to 6; 1 to 1½
3. Remove waste products from blood (or form urine); maintain water balance; maintain electrolyte (or salt) balance; maintain acid-base balance
4. True
5. True
6. False. The autonomic nervous system.
7. True
8. True

Module 12, part 1

1 to 3. See anatomy textbook.
4. Second, sixth

Module 13

1. See anatomy textbook.
2. See anatomy textbook.
3. Events of the normal menstrual cycle are[1]
   a. *Menses* — the breakdown of epithelium via destruction and bursting of endometrial blood vessels and the subsequent sloughing-off process.
   b. *Proliferative stage* — production of estrogen by ovary and repair of uterine surface (occurs simultaneously with ovarian follicular stage and ends with ovulation).
   c. *Secretory stage* — secretion of progesterone by corpus luteum and subsequent thickening of endometrium. This stage ends with cessation of production of progesterone; menses occurs without progesterone support.

[1]Edward J. Reith, et al.: *Textbook of Anatomy and Physiology,* 2d ed., McGraw-Hill, New York, 1978.

Module 15

1 to 3. See anatomy textbook.
4. Cushion; bony surfaces
5. Bursa
6. cervical: concave
   thoracic: convex
   lumbar: concave
7. Cervical and lumbar
8. b
9. Provide means for lengthening of bone (growth)
10. c
11. e

Module 16

1. c
2. Medulla oblongata (brainstem)
3. b
4. Dorsal

5 and 6. See anatomy textbook.

7.
I	h	7
II	d	5
III	b	9, 10
IV	i	8
V	g	4, 15
VI	c	6
VII	a	11, 12
VIII	e	1
IX	l	14
X	j	3
XI	k	13
XII	f	2

8. Cervical 7 and 8
9. False. Pain impulse ascends through the spinothalamic tract on the opposite side of the spinal column.
10. c